Annabel Karmel
Top 100 Meals in Minutes

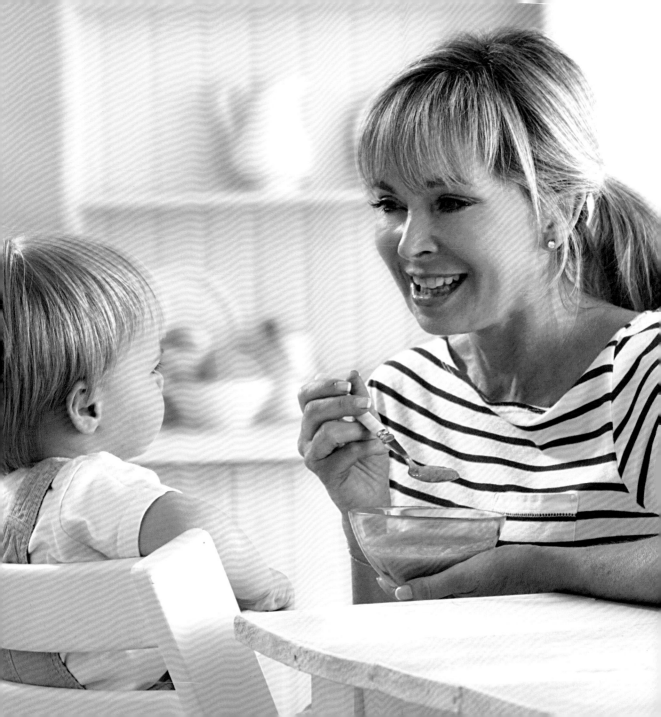

Annabel Karmel
Top 100 Meals in Minutes
Quick and easy meals for babies and toddlers

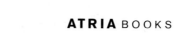

ATRIA BOOKS

New York • London • Toronto • Sydney • New Delhi

To Nicholas, Lara, and Scarlett

ATRIA BOOKS
A Division of Simon & Schuster, Inc.
1230 Avenue of the Americas
New York, NY 10020

Originally published in 2011 by Ebury Press.

First Atria Books hardcover edition December 2014

ATRIA BOOKS and colophon are trademarks of Simon & Schuster, Inc.

For information about special discounts for bulk purchases, please contact Simon
& Schuster Special Sales at 1-866-506-1949 or business@simonandschuster.com.

The Simon & Schuster Speakers Bureau can bring authors to your live event. For
more information or to book an event, contact the Simon & Schuster Speakers
Bureau at 1-866-248-3049 or visit our website at www.simonspeakers.com.

Design: Smith & Gilmour Ltd, London
Photography: Dave King

Manufactured in China

10 9 8 7 6 5 4 3 2 1

Library of Congress Cataloging-in-Publication Data

Karmel, Annabel.
  Top 100 Meals in minutes : quick and easy meals for babies and toddlers /
Annabel Karmel.
     pages   cm
  Includes index.
  1. Infants—Nutrition—Popular works. 2. Toddlers—Nutrition—Popular works.
  3. Quick and easy cooking. I. Title.
  RJ206.K2464   2014
  641.5'622—dc23
                                                      2014009108

ISBN 978-1-4767-2978-7
ISBN 978-1-4767-2980-0 (ebook)

Contents

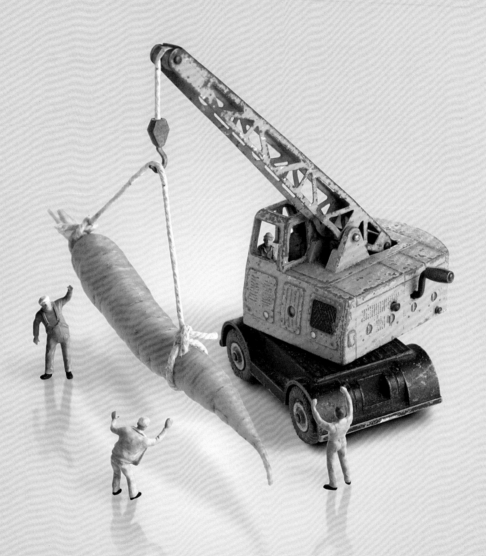

Easy peasy purees and finger foods

Easy peasy purees

There are many purees that don't need any cooking at all. All of these fruit and vegetable purees can be prepared in minutes.

Peach 15

Sweet ripe peaches are delicious and easy to digest. Stir in some baby rice if the puree is too runny.

1 large ripe peach
A little baby rice (optional)

◉ Score a cross with a sharp knife on the base of the peach. Place it in a small bowl and pour boiling water over it.

◉ Drain, then rinse with cold water; the skin should then peel away easily. Cut the flesh away from the pit and mash or puree.

◉ You may want to stir in a little baby rice as it will probably be very runny.

Peach and banana 15

1 small ripe peach
½ small ripe banana

◉ Remove the skin from the peach (as above) and cut the flesh away from the pit. Mash the peach with the banana using a fork, or you could use a hand blender.

◉ Serve on its own or mixed with a little baby rice.

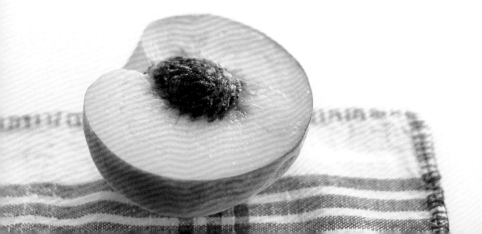

Mango 5

Known as the "King of Fruit," mangoes are rich in antioxidants—rich health boosters.

½ medium ripe mango

◉ Remove the skin from the mango and cut the flesh into cubes.

◉ Mash or puree using a hand blender until smooth.

Mango and banana 5

½ small ripe mango
½ small ripe banana

◉ Prepare the mango as for the mango puree.

◉ Slice the banana.

◉ Mash the banana and mango, or puree using a hand blender.

Mango and strawberry 5

½ small ripe mango
2 strawberries

◉ Prepare the mango as in the mango puree.

◉ Blend the mango flesh with the strawberries.

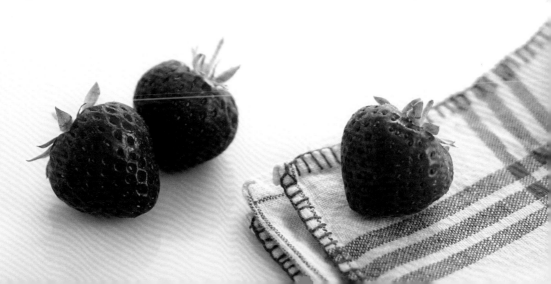

Apple, strawberry, and banana

15

Strawberries are rich in vitamin C and have a natural sweetness, which makes this delicious.

SUITABLE FOR FREEZING
SUITABLE FROM 6 MONTHS
MAKES 3 PORTIONS
2 apples, peeled and diced (about 1¼ cups)
5 medium strawberries, quartered
½ small banana

◉ Put all the ingredients in a saucepan and cook over low heat for about 8 minutes, or until the apples are tender, then puree with a hand blender.

Pear, apple, and blueberry

15

Blueberries contain more antioxidants than any other fruits.

SUITABLE FOR FREEZING
SUITABLE FROM 6 MONTHS
MAKES 3 PORTIONS
2 ripe pears, peeled
2 apples, peeled
2 to 3 tablespoons water
¾ cup blueberries

◉ Remove the cores from the pears and apples. Coarsely chop them and place in a saucepan with the water and blueberries.

◉ Simmer for 8 to 10 minutes, until soft. Whiz until smooth, using a hand blender.

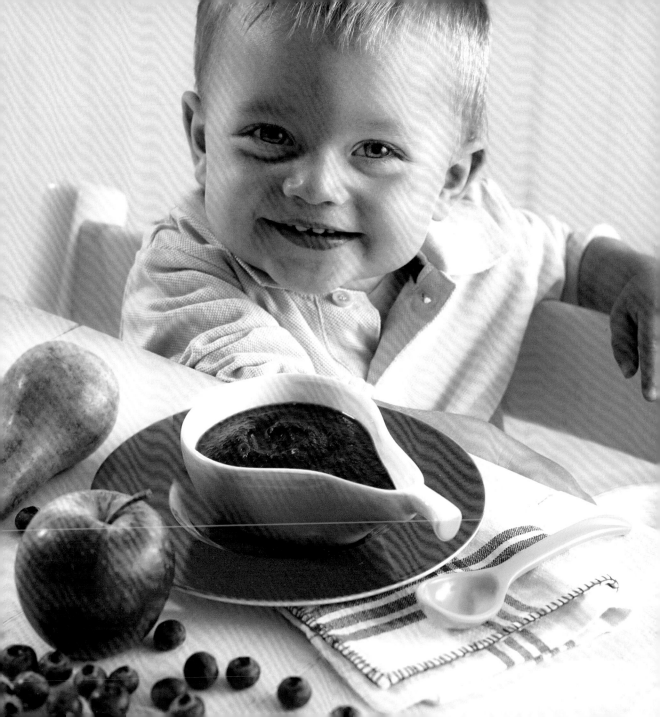

Plum 10

Always make sure that you taste the fruit before giving it to your baby. Some plums can be quite sour, but sweet ones are delicious.

SUITABLE FOR FREEZING
SUITABLE FROM 6 MONTHS
MAKES 1 PORTION
2 large plums
Baby rice, crumbled zwieback, mashed banana (optional)

◉ Peel the plums in the same way as you did the peach (see page 8). Chop the flesh.

◉ Puree the plums uncooked if ripe and juicy, or steam them for a few minutes until tender. They are good mixed with baby rice, crumbled zwieback, or mashed banana.

Peach and blueberry 15

You could use nectarines instead of peaches. Sweet white nectarines are especially good.

SUITABLE FOR FREEZING
SUITABLE FROM 6 MONTHS
MAKES 2 PORTIONS
2 medium ripe peaches
⅓ cup blueberries

◉ Peel the peaches, remove the pits, and cut into chunks.

◉ Put into a saucepan with the blueberries and cook for 3 minutes over medium heat.

◉ Blend to a puree.

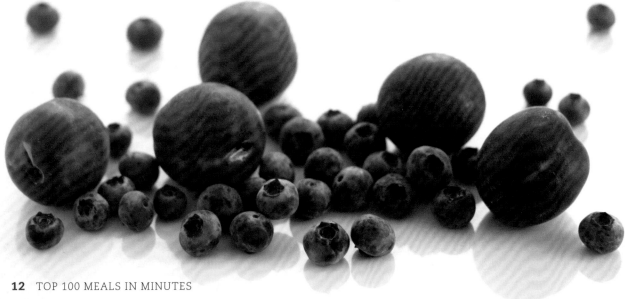

Banana 5

Banana makes perfect portable baby food as it comes in its own packaging. Banana is good for the treatment of both diarrhea and constipation.

NOT SUITABLE FOR FREEZING
SUITABLE FROM 6 MONTHS
MAKES 1 PORTION
½ small banana
A little breast or formula milk (optional)

◉ Mash the banana with a fork. During the first stages of weaning add a little of your baby's usual milk, if necessary, to thin out the consistency and provide a familiar taste.

Papaya 5

Papaya is rich in vitamin C and beta-carotene. Papaya is also high in soluble fiber, which is important for normal bowel function.

NOT SUITABLE FOR FREEZING
SUITABLE FROM 6 MONTHS
MAKES 1 PORTION
½ small ripe papaya

◉ Remove the seeds, scoop out the flesh, and mash or puree until smooth.

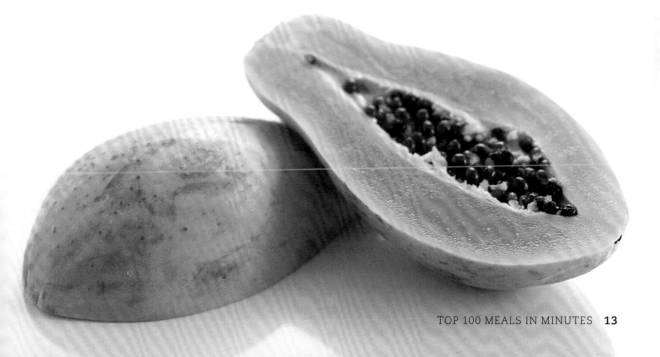

Avocado 5

Avocados contain more nutrients than any other fruit. They are rich in vitamin E, which boosts the immune system. They are also rich in monounsaturated fat, the good type of fat. Babies need nutrient-dense foods, and the high-calorie content of avocados makes them ideal for growing babies.

NOT SUITABLE FOR FREEZING
SUITABLE FROM 6 MONTHS
MAKES 1 PORTION
½ small ripe avocado
A little breast or formula milk (optional)

◉ Remove the pit. Scoop out the flesh and mash together with a little of your baby's usual milk.

Avocado and banana 5

This is a popular combination.

NOT SUITABLE FOR FREEZING
SUITABLE FROM 6 MONTHS
MAKES 1 PORTION
½ small ripe avocado
½ small ripe banana
1 to 2 tablespoons breast or formula milk

◉ Remove the avocado pit and mash the avocado and banana together. If you like, stir in a little of your baby's usual milk.

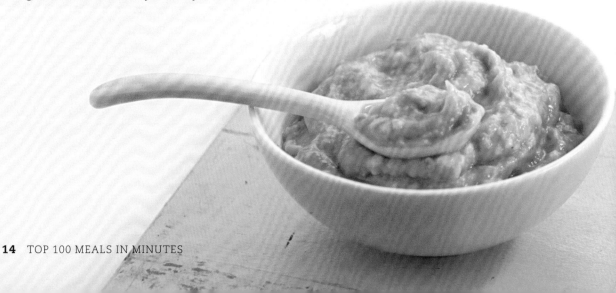

Sweet potato, carrot, and corn

Some vegetables, such as sweet potato, carrot, butternut squash, pumpkin, and corn are naturally sweet and popular with babies. Orange root vegetables are also rich in beta-carotene, which is essential for growth, healthy skin, and fighting infection.

1 medium sweet potato, peeled and diced (about 1⅔ cups)

1 medium carrot, chopped (about ½ cup)

2 tablespoons corn, fresh, canned, or frozen (thawed)

◉ Put the sweet potato and carrot into a steamer and cook for about 15 minutes, or until tender.

◉ Puree the sweet potato and carrot with the corn and ¼ cup of the water from the bottom of the steamer.

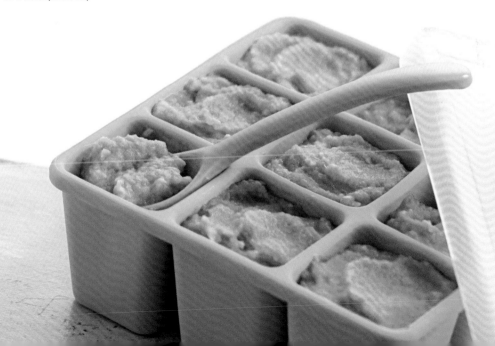

Lovely lentil puree

You might not have thought of giving your baby lentils, but some of my most popular baby recipes are lentil purees. Lentils are a good source of protein, iron, and fiber. They are good for all babies and especially good to include in your baby's diet if you are a vegetarian.

1 tablespoon canola oil
¼ cup finely chopped onion
2 medium carrots, diced (about ¾ cup)
2 tablespoons chopped celery
⅓ cup split red lentils, rinsed
1 medium sweet potato, peeled and diced (about 1⅔ cups)
1¼ cups sodium-free vegetable broth or water
⅓ cup grated Cheddar cheese

◉ Heat the oil in a saucepan. Add the onion, carrots, and celery and sauté for about 5 minutes, or until softened.

◉ Add the lentils and sauté for 1 minute. Stir in the sweet potato and add the broth.

◉ Bring to a boil, reduce the heat, and simmer covered for about 20 minutes, or until the lentils are soft.

◉ Puree in a blender and stir in the cheese until melted.

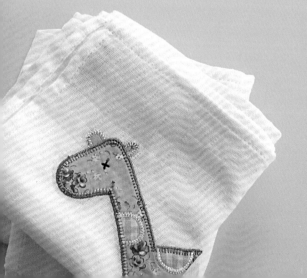

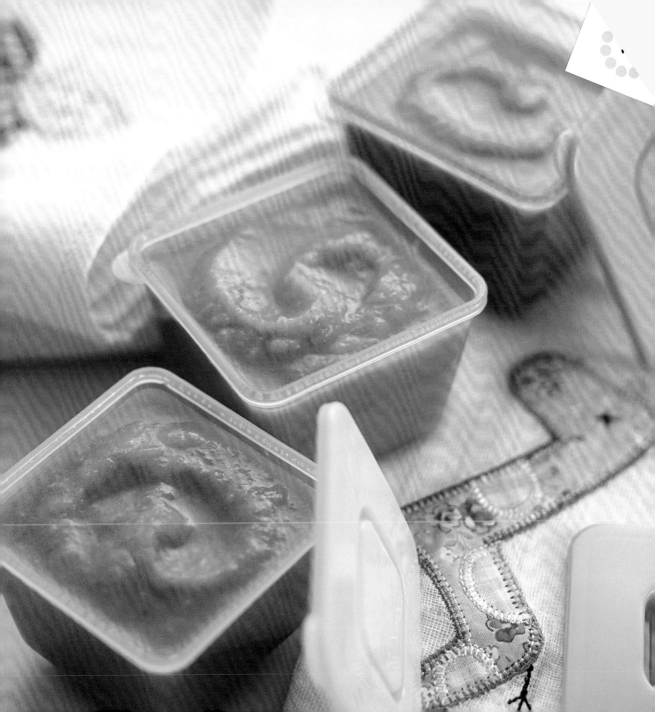

Lentil and vegetable puree

A tasty puree with nutritious ingredients where I have sped up the cooking process by using lentils in a can. Lentils are a good non-meat source of iron. It is important to introduce solids at six months because the iron a baby inherits from his or her mother runs out at this age.

1 tablespoon olive oil
¼ cup finely chopped leek
⅓ cup finely chopped carrot
½ garlic clove, crushed
½ cup drained canned lentils, rinsed
1 cup canned diced tomatoes
7 tablespoons water
1 teaspoon tomato paste
1 small bay leaf
1 apricot, chopped
1 tablespoon chopped fresh basil
2 tablespoons plain yogurt
   (whole milk)

◉ Heat the oil in a saucepan. Add the leek, carrot, and garlic. Sauté for 5 minutes.

◉ Add the lentils, tomatoes, water, tomato paste, bay leaf, and apricot. Bring to a boil. Cover and simmer for 8 to 10 minutes.

◉ Whiz with a hand blender until smooth. Stir in the basil and yogurt.

Mashed sweet potato with spinach

A good way to introduce stronger-tasting green vegetables is to mix them together with sweet-tasting root vegetables. Low-fat dairy products are not suitable for children under two as they need the calories to fuel their rapid growth.

1 cup peeled and diced sweet
   potato
¾ cup peeled and diced potato
¾ cup boiling water
1½ cups fresh baby spinach
¼ cup frozen peas
½ cup grated Cheddar cheese
1 tablespoon milk

◉ Put the sweet potato and potato into a pan, cover with boiling water and cook, covered, for 10 minutes.

◉ Add the spinach and peas, cover and cook for 3 minutes. Uncover and, if any liquid is still left, cook a little longer.

◉ Stir in the cheese and milk, then whiz until smooth, using a hand blender.

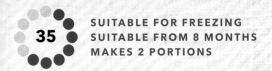
Pasta shells with butternut squash and tomato sauce

This fresh tomato sauce is very tasty and, because it has butternut squash and cheese blended into it, it is more nutritious than an ordinary tomato sauce.

1 cup peeled and diced butternut
   squash
¼ cup mini shell pasta
3 medium tomatoes
1 tablespoon butter
⅓ cup grated Cheddar cheese

◉ Steam the butternut squash for 10 minutes, or until tender.

◉ Cook the pasta following the package directions.

◉ Cut a cross in the base of the tomatoes using a sharp knife. Put them in a bowl and cover with boiling water. Leave for 1 minute. Drain and rinse with cold water. The skin should peel off easily. Cut the tomatoes into quarters and remove the seeds.

◉ Melt the butter in a small saucepan. Add the tomatoes and sauté until mushy. Stir in the cheese until melted.

◉ Blend the butternut squash with the tomato and cheese sauce. Drain the pasta and stir into the sauce.

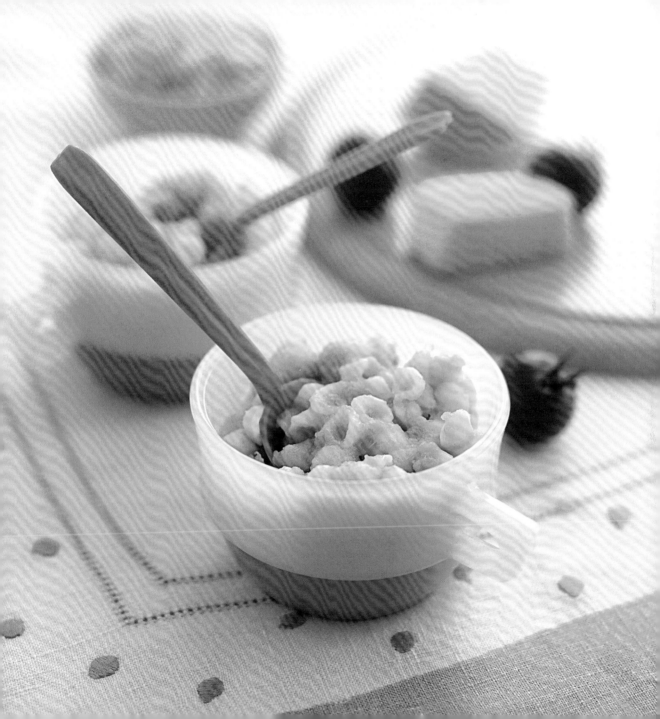

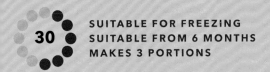
Poached salmon with sweet potato and peas

It's hard to find a jar of baby food that contains oily fish such as salmon, yet the essential fatty acids in oily fish are particularly important for the development of your baby's brain, nervous system, and vision. Fats like these are a major component of the brain; for this reason 50 percent of the calories in breast milk are composed of fat.

⅓ cup vegetable broth or water
¾ cup peeled and diced
  sweet potato
4 ounces salmon fillet, skin
  removed, cut into ⅜ inch-cubes
2 tablespoons frozen peas
½ cup grated sharp Cheddar cheese

◉ Put the broth in a saucepan with the sweet potato. Bring to a boil, then cook over medium heat for 7 to 8 minutes, or until the sweet potato is just tender.

◉ Add the salmon and peas, cover again, and simmer for 3 to 4 minutes, until the fish flakes easily and the vegetables are tender.

◉ Remove from the heat and stir in the cheese. Blend to a puree for young babies or mash for children on lumpy foods.

◉ Cool as quickly as possible, then cover and chill. You can freeze individual portions, thaw overnight in the fridge, then reheat until piping hot. Stir and let cool slightly before serving.

Cod with sweet potato

If you want your baby to enjoy eating fish, then introduce it early. You can give them fish from six months. Begin with mildly flavored white fish such as cod or pollock with a favorite vegetable puree or a cheese sauce.

Pat of butter
½ cup finely chopped onion
1 cup peeled and diced sweet potato
⅔ cup milk
1 small bay leaf
4 ounces cod fillet, skin removed, cut into 2 inch-pieces

◉ Melt the butter in a saucepan. Add the onion and sauté for 5 minutes, until nearly soft.

◉ Add the sweet potato, milk, and bay leaf. Bring to a boil, cover and simmer for 10 minutes, until the sweet potato is tender.

◉ Add the cod and cook for another 2 to 3 minutes. Remove the bay leaf, then whiz using a hand blender to make a fine puree. You can mash for children on lumpier foods.

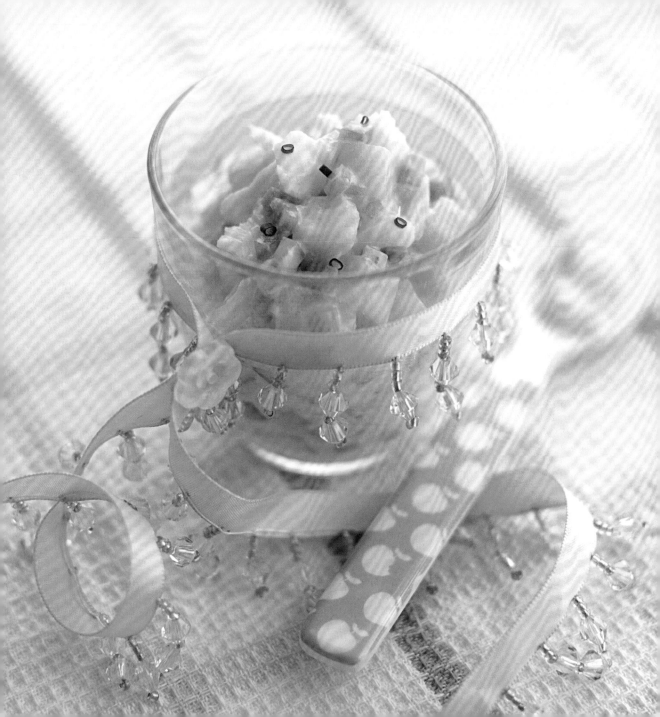

Cherub's chowder

Fats from dairy products such as butter, cheese, yogurt, and milk are fine for babies as they provide vitamins A and D. It is not good just to give babies fruit and vegetable purees, since they are low in calories.

Pat of butter
1 small celery stalk, finely diced
1 small leek, coarsely chopped
1 small carrot, finely diced
¾ cup peeled and finely diced
   potato
1 tablespoon all-purpose flour
1⅓ cups milk
2 tablespoons grated Parmesan
   cheese
½ teaspoon Dijon mustard
4 ounces cod or haddock,
   skin removed, cut into
   ¾ inch-cubes
1 tablespoon chopped fresh chives
½ teaspoon lemon juice

◉ Melt the butter in a saucepan. Add the celery, leek, carrot, and potato. Coat in the butter and gently sauté for 3 to 4 minutes. Sprinkle with the flour.

◉ Add the milk and stir until blended. Bring to a boil, stirring until thickened. Cover and simmer for 8 minutes, until the vegetables are cooked.

◉ Add the cheese, mustard, and cod and continue to simmer for 5 minutes, until the cod is cooked through. Stir in the chives and lemon juice.

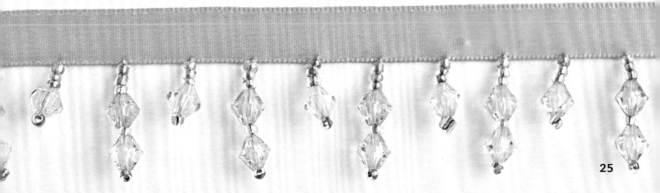

Baby's first fish pie

Although you should continue with formula or breast milk for the entire first year, whole cow's milk can be used in cooking and with cereals from six months.

SUITABLE FOR FREEZING
SUITABLE FROM 6 MONTHS
MAKES 4 PORTIONS

1⅓ cups peeled and diced potatoes
1 small onion, finely diced
¾ cup milk
7 tablespoons low-sodium fish broth
⅓ cup frozen peas
6 ounces cod, skin removed, cut into small cubes
1 teaspoon lemon juice
3 tablespoon grated Parmesan cheese
1 teaspoon fresh chopped dill

◉ Put the potatoes and onion into a saucepan. Cover with the milk and broth. Bring to a boil, cover, and simmer for 10 minutes.

◉ Add the peas and cod and continue to cook for 5 minutes.

◉ Whiz to a puree in a blender. Add the lemon juice, cheese, and dill.

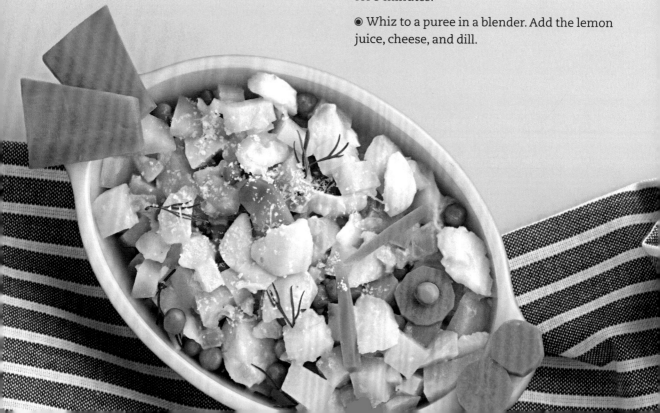

Salmon smash

As your baby gets older you can mash rather than puree the food. This is a delicious combination of mashed potatoes, carrot, and broccoli with flaked salmon. The healthy fats found in oily fish encourage growth as well as the development of your baby's brain, nervous system, and vision.

SUITABLE FOR FREEZING
SUITABLE FROM 7 MONTHS
MAKES 3 PORTIONS
1½ cups peeled and diced potatoes
1 small carrot, peeled and diced
⅔ cup broccoli florets
3 ounces salmon fillet
1 tablespoon butter
¼ cup milk
½ cup grated Cheddar cheese

◉ Put the potatoes and carrot into a saucepan. Cover with boiling water and cook for 15 minutes, or until tender.

◉ Meanwhile, steam the broccoli for about 6 minutes, until tender. Cook the salmon either by poaching it in milk or broth until it flakes easily with a fork, or put it into a microwave dish, dot with one third of the butter. Cover, leaving an air vent, and cook for about 1½ minutes.

◉ Mash the potatoes, carrot, and broccoli with the remaining butter, milk, and cheese. Flake the salmon and stir into the mash.

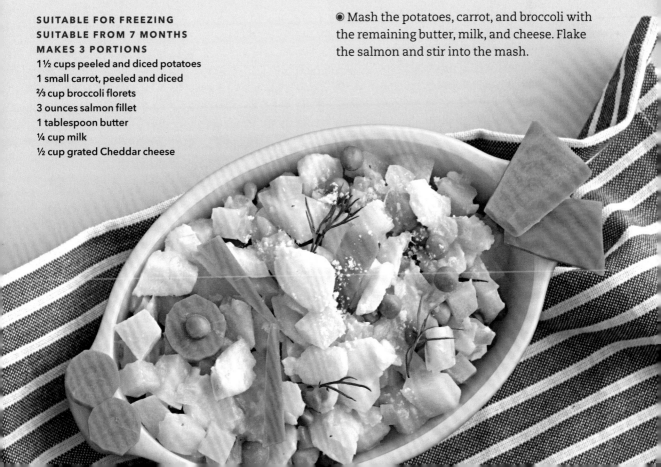

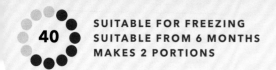
Chicken with butternut squash and tarragon

Since you can't add salt to baby purees, it's a good idea to add fresh herbs to bring out the flavor.

Pat of butter
½ cup finely chopped onion
¾ cup peeled and diced butternut
   squash
4 ounces chicken breast
   cut into small pieces
1 tablespoon all-purpose flour
7 tablespoons milk
⅛ teaspoon lemon zest
1 teaspoon lemon juice
1 tablespoon finely grated
   Parmesan cheese
⅛ teaspoon finely chopped
   fresh tarragon

◉ Melt the butter in a saucepan. Add the onion and sauté for 5 minutes, until softened.

◉ Add the butternut squash and chicken and fry for 1 to 2 minutes.

◉ Sprinkle with the flour, then blend in the milk. Bring to a boil, stirring until slightly thickened.

◉ Add the lemon zest and juice, cover, and simmer for 10 minutes, until the squash is soft and the chicken is cooked.

◉ Puree using a hand blender, then stir in the cheese and tarragon.

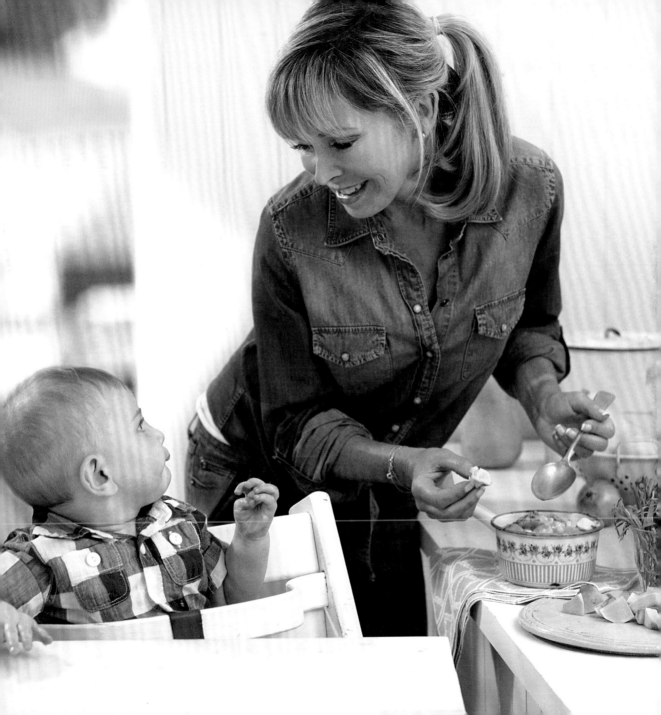

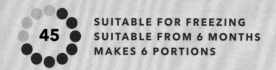
Chicken with carrot and apple

When my son was a baby, he refused to eat chicken until I combined it with apple, which he loved.

1 tablespoon canola oil
⅓ cup finely chopped leek
2 tablespoons finely chopped celery
½ cup diced carrot
1 garlic clove, crushed
4 ounces chicken cut into chunks
1¾ cups peeled and diced sweet
   potatoes
½ cup peeled and chopped apple
1 cup boiling low-sodium chicken
   broth or water
1 sprig fresh thyme

◉ Heat the oil in a saucepan and sauté the leek for 2 minutes.

◉ Add the celery and carrot and cook for 5 minutes. Add the garlic and sauté for 1 minute.

◉ Stir in the chicken and sauté for 2 to 3 minutes, or until the chicken is cooked.

◉ Add the sweet potatoes and apple and pour in the chicken broth. Add the thyme sprig. Cover and cook over low heat for 20 minutes.

◉ Remove the thyme sprig and blitz to a puree.

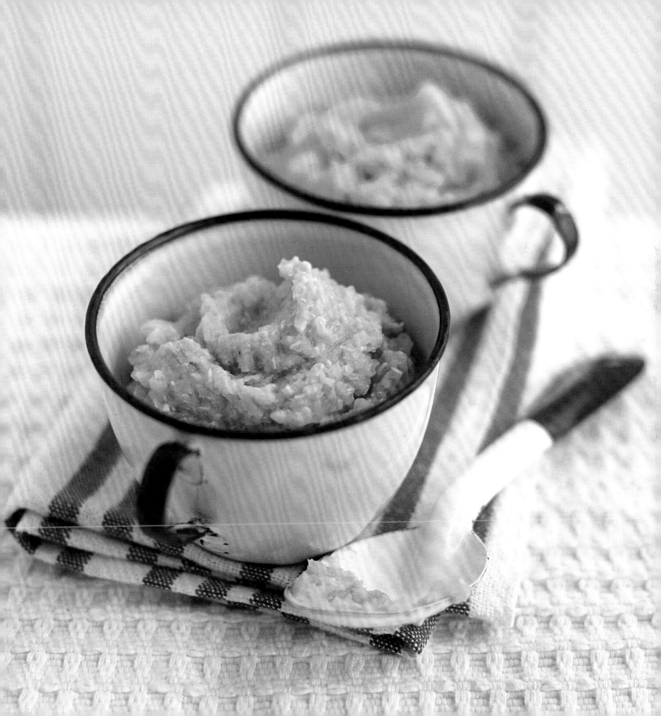

Creamy chicken with sweet potato 20

A tasty recipe to make with cooked chicken.

SUITABLE FOR FREEZING
SUITABLE FROM 6 MONTHS
MAKES 2 PORTIONS
¾ cup peeled and diced sweet potato
1 tablespoon butter
1 tablespoon all-purpose flour
⅔ cup milk
2 tablespoons grated Cheddar cheese
¼ cup diced cooked chicken

◉ Steam the sweet potato for about 10 minutes, or until tender.

◉ Melt the butter in a small saucepan, stir in the flour to make a roux, then gradually stir in the milk.

◉ Bring to a boil, then reduce the heat, and cook for a couple of minutes. Remove from the heat and stir in the cheese until melted.

◉ Whiz the sweet potato with the chicken and cheese sauce.

California chicken 30

Avocados contain more nutrients than any other fruit. They are also rich in monounsaturated fat, the good type of fat that helps prevent heart disease.

NOT SUITABLE FOR FREEZING
SUITABLE FROM 6 MONTHS
MAKES 1 PORTION
¼ cup diced cooked chicken
½ small avocado
2 tablespoon plain yogurt (whole milk)
1 tablespoon grated Swiss cheese

◉ Blend all the ingredients together.

Chicken with tomato and sweet pepper

Adding pure apple juice and sweet potato makes this puree appealing to babies, and stirring in the cream cheese gives it a slightly creamier texture.

1 tablespoon olive oil
½ cup finely diced red bell pepper
⅓ cup peeled and diced
   sweet potato
4 ounces chicken breast,
   cut into ¾-inch pieces
½ small garlic clove, crushed
½ cup diced tomatoes
⅓ cup apple juice
1 tablespoon cream cheese

◉ Heat the oil in a saucepan. Add the bell pepper and sweet potato and sauté for 5 minutes.

◉ Add the chicken and garlic and fry for 1 minute. Add the tomatoes and apple juice.

◉ Bring to a boil. Cover and simmer for 8 to 10 minutes, until soft.

◉ Whiz using a hand blender until smooth. Stir in the cream cheese.

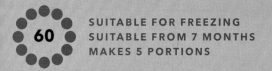

SUITABLE FOR FREEZING
SUITABLE FROM 7 MONTHS
MAKES 5 PORTIONS

Beef and carrot casserole

The most easily absorbed source of iron is red meat. Iron is important for your baby's brain development, especially between six months and two years. The iron a baby inherits from its mother runs out at around six months.

7 ounces ground beef (lean)
1 small onion, finely chopped
2 small carrots, coarsely chopped
1 celery stalk, finely diced
1 tablespoon all-purpose flour
3 tablespoons apple juice
¾ cup sodium-free beef broth
½ cup sodium-free tomato sauce
1 teaspoon tomato paste
½ teaspoon dried thyme
Dash of Worcestershire sauce
 (optional)
1 tablespoon grated Parmesan
 cheese

◉ Heat a saucepan and brown the beef, then add the onion, carrots, and celery.

◉ Fry over medium heat for 3 to 4 minutes until lightly browned. Sprinkle with the flour. Blend in the apple juice, broth, and tomato sauce.

◉ Bring to a boil and add the tomato paste and thyme. Cover and simmer for 30 minutes, until tender.

◉ Add the Worcestershire sauce, if using, and the Parmesan. Blend to a puree for young babies.

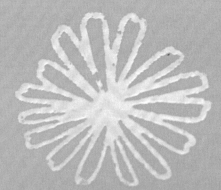

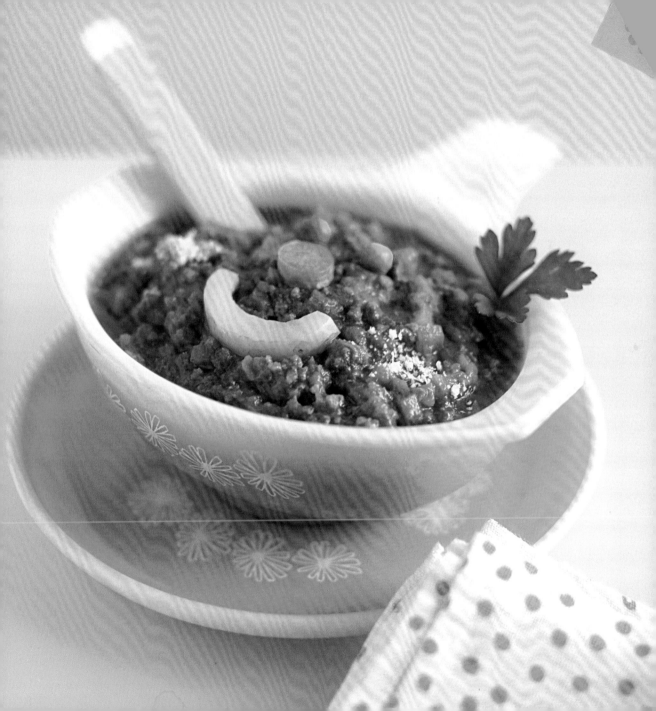

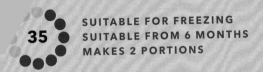

Beef with sweet pepper and tomato puree

This is my baby version of meat and two veggies. Don't delay feeding your baby meat much beyond six months as it provides the best source of iron.

1 tablespoon olive oil
½ cup finely chopped red onion
¼ cup finely diced red bell pepper
2 ounces top loin steak,
    sliced into small thin strips
⅛ teaspoon ground coriander
1 cup canned diced tomatoes
2 teaspoons apple juice

◉ Heat the oil in a saucepan. Add the onion and bell pepper, and sauté for 5 minutes, until nearly soft.

◉ Add the steak and coriander and fry for 2 minutes. Add the tomatoes and apple juice. Cover and simmer for 10 minutes.

◉ Puree using a hand blender until completely smooth.

Cheesy pasta with broccoli and peas

This is a good way to encourage your baby to enjoy greens.

Pat of butter
1 small leek, white and pale green
   parts, finely chopped
1 tablespoon all-purpose flour
1 cup milk
½ cup grated Cheddar cheese
¼ teaspoon Dijon mustard
⅓ cup small pasta shapes
⅓ cup very small broccoli florets
⅓ cup frozen baby peas

◉ Melt the butter in a saucepan. Add the leek and sauté for 2 to 3 minutes, until soft. Sprinkle with the flour, then blend in the milk. Bring to a boil, stirring until thickened.

◉ Add the cheese and mustard. Cook the pasta in boiling water following the package directions.

◉ Add the broccoli to the pasta 5 minutes before the end of the cooking time and cook for 2 minutes. Add the peas and cook for 3 to 4 minutes. Drain and mix the pasta with the sauce.

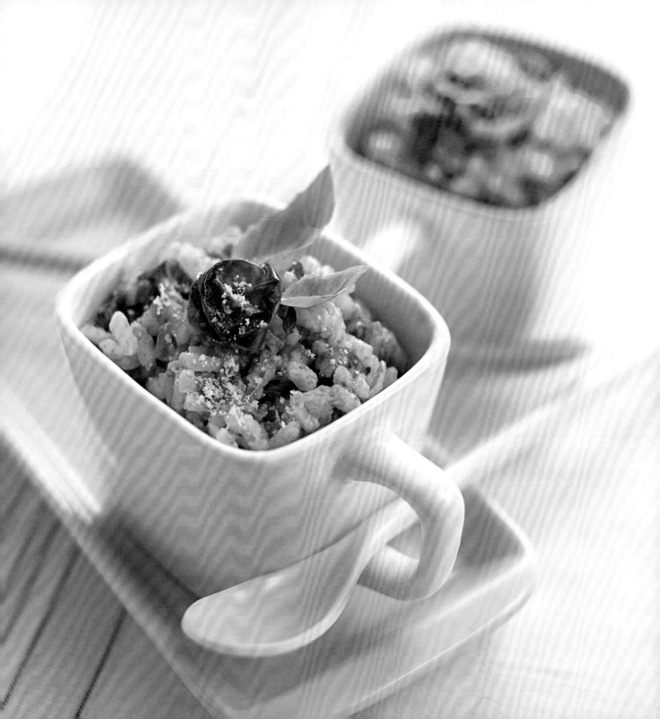

Risotto with tomato and basil

Making a risotto is a good way to introduce texture to a baby's diet.

1 teaspoon olive oil
1 onion, finely chopped
1 leek, white and pale green parts,
   finely chopped
1 garlic clove, crushed
½ cup long-grain rice
1¼ cups water
⅓ cup grated Parmesan cheese
3 tomatoes, seeded and chopped
2 tablespoons finely chopped fresh
   basil

◉ Heat the oil in a saucepan. Add the onion and leek and sauté for 2 to 3 minutes. Add the garlic and fry for 30 seconds.

◉ Add the rice and coat it in the onion mixture. Pour in the water. Bring to a boil.

◉ Cover, reduce the heat, and simmer for 15 to 20 minutes, or until all the water is absorbed and the rice is cooked.

◉ Add the Parmesan, tomatoes, and basil. Gently mix together.

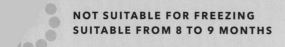

First finger foods

Finger foods need to be fairly simple and slightly soft. So until your baby can chew properly, to avoid the risk of choking, give steamed vegetables rather than raw, and soft fruits. Also take care not to give any foods your baby might choke on such as whole grapes or fruits with pits.

Fruits

Start with soft fruits such as banana, pear, peach, plum, mango, peeled halved grapes, or dried apricot, and then move on to apple.

Vegetables

Start with steamed vegetables such as carrot sticks, broccoli and cauliflower florets. From four years of age, you can move on to raw vegetables such as cucumber, carrot, and bell pepper sticks.

● ● ● ● ● ● ● ● ● ● ● ● ●
TIP
It is often better to give large pieces of fruit or vegetables, which your child can hold and eat rather than bite-size pieces.

OTHER GOOD FINGER FOODS

◉ Sticks of cheese

◉ Dried fruits, such as apricot or apple

◉ Rice cakes

◉ Pita bread

◉ Bagels

◉ Dry cereals, but avoid the sugar-coated variety

◉ Toast sticks spread with peanut butter, cream cheese, pure fruit spread

◉ Sticks of grilled cheese

◉ Mini popsicles made from fresh fruit or fruit juice (good for sore gums)

Sandwiches

Sandwiches make good finger food, and for little ones it is best not to have too much bread or too much filling. It can be a good idea to flatten the bread a little with a rolling pin so that it is easier for small children to handle.

Presentation is important. A child is far more likely to eat something that looks appealing. Try cutting sandwiches into shapes using cookie cutters or use one slice of white and one slice of whole wheat bread to make sandwiches. Remove the crusts and cut into squares, then turn alternate squares over so that you have a checkerboard sandwich.

HERE ARE SOME FAVORITE SANDWICH FILLINGS TO TRY

◉ Hummus and finely grated carrot

◉ Mashed tuna mixed with mayonnaise and a little ketchup

◉ Cream cheese and grated cucumber

◉ Thinly sliced cheese and ham

◉ Thinly sliced cheese and tomato (remove the seeds so that the bread doesn't become too soggy)

◉ Cream cheese mixed with a little maple syrup and then a layer of mashed banana

◉ Hard-boiled egg mashed with a little mayonnaise and alfalfa sprouts

◉ Edamame hummus with shredded lettuce

◉ Smoked salmon and cream cheese

◉ Tuna with corn, scallion, and mayonnaise

◉ Mashed canned sardines with ketchup

◉ Peanut butter and mashed banana

◉ Peanut butter and low-sugar strawberry jam

◉ Cream cheese and raspberry jam

◉ Cream cheese and chopped dried apricot

◉ Chopped chicken with mayonnaise, corn, and scallion

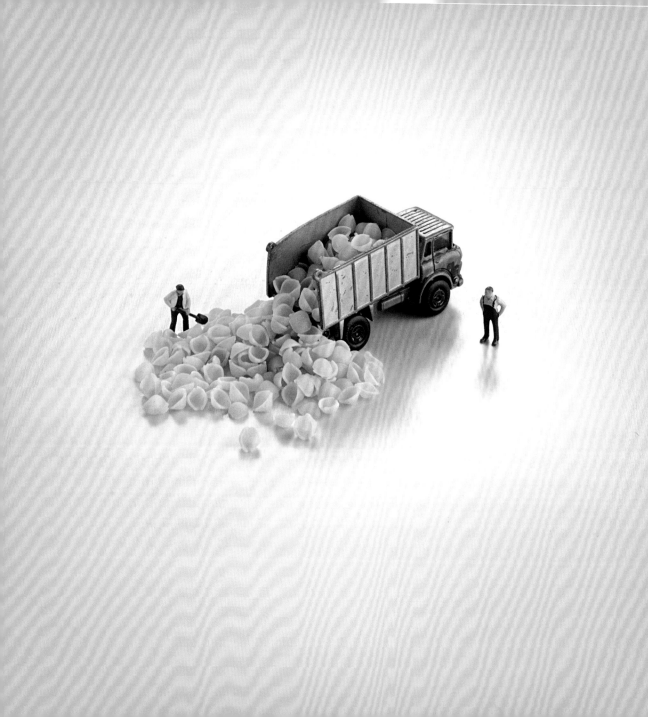

Pronto pasta

Fresh tomato sauce with sun-dried tomatoes

This is a good sauce to make when you have some tasty ripe tomatoes on hand. Some markets sell oven-dried tomatoes, which would be delicious in the sauce too.

1 tablespoon olive oil
1 small onion, finely chopped
1 large garlic clove, crushed
1 pound ripe tomatoes, chopped
Pinch of sugar
¼ teaspoon balsamic vinegar
8 ounces small penne pasta
4 sun-dried tomatoes (packed in oil), chopped

◉ To make the sauce, heat the oil in a saucepan and add the onion and simmer for 10 minutes until soft. Then add the garlic and fry for 1 minute. Add the tomatoes and sugar. Season to taste.

◉ Bring to a boil, then sauté for 10 to 15 minutes, until the tomatoes have broken down. Whiz the sauce with a hand blender until smooth, then add the vinegar.

◉ Cook the pasta in boiling salted water until it is tender. Drain, toss with the sauce, and mix in the sun-dried tomatoes.

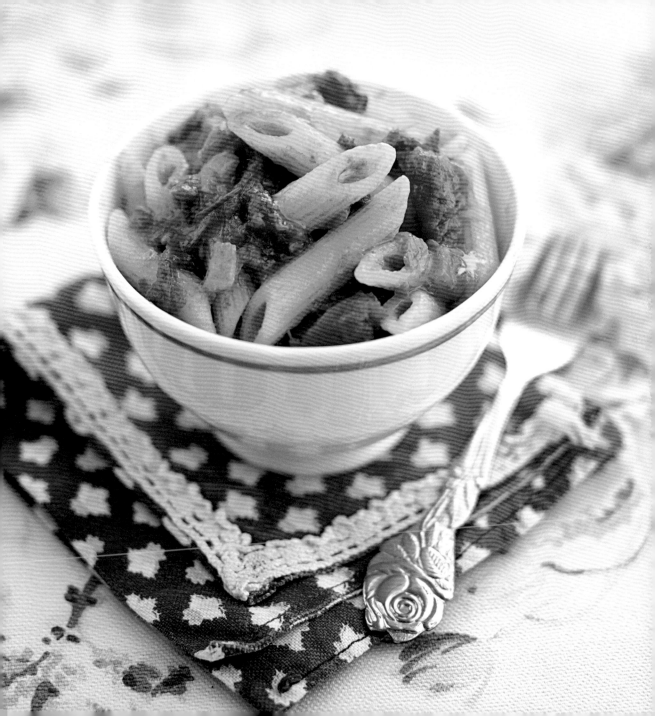

Tomato and mascarpone sauce with penne

This makes a lovely creamy tomato sauce, with the mascarpone stirred in.
If you don't have mascarpone you could use cream cheese instead.

1 tablespoon olive oil
3 scallions, thinly sliced
1 garlic clove, crushed
1 (14-ounce) can diced tomatoes
3 sun-dried tomatoes (packed
   in oil), chopped
2 tablespoons tomato paste
2 tablespoons ketchup
1½ teaspoons sugar
8 ounces penne pasta
¼ cup mascarpone
Salt and pepper

Optional to serve
Parmesan cheese, grated
4 large basil leaves, shredded

◉ Heat the oil in a deep frying pan and sauté the scallions and garlic for 1 minute. Add all the tomato ingredients plus the sugar, bring to a boil and cook for 15 minutes until very thick (in a wok it may take slightly longer). Meanwhile, cook the pasta following the package directions.

◉ Transfer the sauce to a blender, or bowl, and cool slightly, then add the mascarpone and blend in the blender, or with a hand blender, until smooth. Season to taste.

◉ Reserve a cupful of the cooking water before draining the pasta. Return the pasta to the saucepan and toss with the sauce, adding 2 to 3 tablespoons of the cooking water if the pasta becomes too dry. Spoon onto plates and serve with the Parmesan and perhaps some fresh basil, if your child likes it.

Spaghetti with pesto

If you are making pesto in advance, make it with 7 tablespoons of the oil. Transfer to a container and pour the remaining 3 tablespoons of oil over the surface. This will stop the pesto from turning dark. Store in the fridge for up to one week and stir before using. Pesto also freezes well in airtight containers for up to three months.

½ cup pine nuts
2 cups (loosely packed)
   fresh basil leaves
1 large garlic clove
⅔ cup extra-virgin olive oil
½ cup grated Parmesan cheese
10 ounces spaghetti
Salt and pepper

◉ Toast the pine nuts for 2 to 3 minutes in a dry frying pan (or buy toasted pine nuts), then leave to cool.

◉ Transfer them to a food processor. Add the basil and garlic and whiz until everything is finely chopped. Then pour in the oil through the funnel, with the motor running, until combined.

◉ Add the Parmesan and season to taste before pulsing 4 to 5 times to combine. Spoon into a bowl.

◉ Cook the pasta following the package directions. Before draining, reserve a cupful of the cooking water. Mix the pasta with the pesto and add a little cooking water if the pasta gets too dry. Transfer to plates and serve with extra Parmesan.

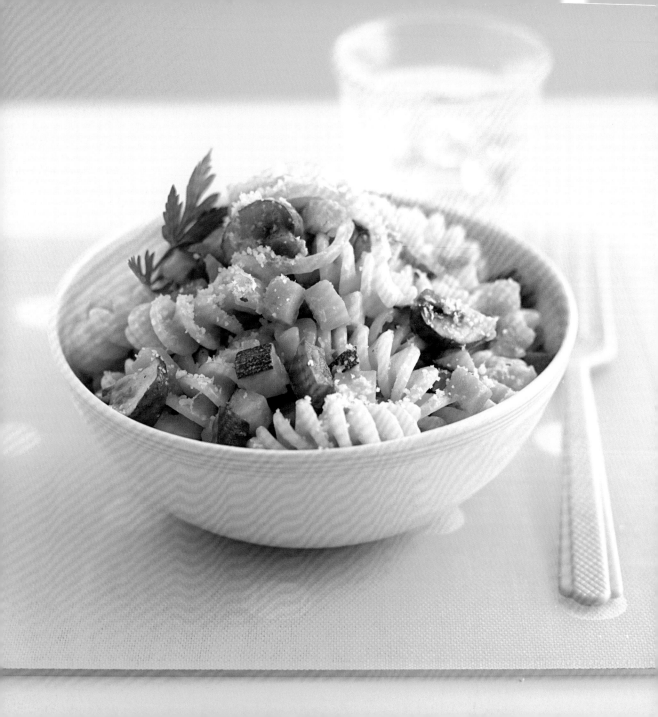

Pasta primavera

Combining diced vegetables with pasta is a great way to get fussy eaters to have more vegetables in their diet. Simply mix the crème fraîche, broth, and Parmesan to make a quick, tasty, light cheese sauce.

6 ounces fusilli pasta
2 tablespoons canola oil
1 small onion, sliced
1 cup peeled and diced butternut
   squash
½ red bell pepper, diced
1 medium zucchini, diced
   (about ¾ cup)
1½ cups sliced cremini mushrooms
1 garlic clove, crushed
⅔ cup vegetable broth
⅓ cup crème fraîche or heavy cream
⅔ cup grated Parmesan cheese
2 tablespoons chopped fresh basil
Pinch of salt

◉ Cook the pasta following the package directions and drain.

◉ Heat the oil in a frying pan on medium-low heat. Add the onion and butternut squash and gently fry for 5 minutes. Add the remaining vegetables and fry for 3 minutes. Add the garlic and fry for 1 minute.

◉ Add the broth to the pan and let it bubble away until it has reduced by half.

◉ Finally, add the crème fraîche, cheese, and basil, then season with a little salt and toss together with the pasta.

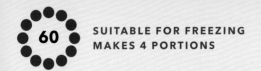

Spinach and tuna lasagna

To save time, you can use store-bought marinara sauce to make this tasty lasagna. Make sure the top of the lasagna is completely covered with sauce so that the pasta doesn't burn.

1 tablespoon olive oil
1 onion, chopped
1 garlic clove, crushed
10 cups fresh spinach, washed
⅔ cup cream cheese
1 (12-ounce) can tuna in water, drained
Salt and pepper
2 cups store-bought marinara sauce
3 large sheets fresh lasagna (about 6 ounces) or 6 small sheets
4 ounces fresh mozzarella, thinly sliced
2 to 3 tablespoons grated Parmesan cheese

⊚ Preheat the oven to 400°F. Heat the oil in a wok or large frying pan and sauté the onion for 5 to 6 minutes, until soft.

⊚ Add the garlic and spinach and sauté 3 to 4 minutes more, until the spinach has thoroughly wilted. If your child is fussy you may want to coarsely chop the spinach and onion mixture in a food processor, then return to the pan.

⊚ Add the cream cheese and stir until melted, then stir in the drained tuna and season to taste.

⊚ Spread a thick layer of tomato sauce in the bottom of a baking dish (about 8 x 8 inches). Put a layer of lasagna on the sauce (trim the sheets to fit the dish, if necessary), then spread half the tuna mixture on top. Spoon over a quarter of the tomato sauce, spreading it out slightly, then add another layer of pasta, tuna, and a quarter more of the sauce.

⊚ Top with a third layer of pasta and spread with the remaining tomato sauce. Cover with the mozzarella and sprinkle with the Parmesan.

⊚ Bake for 40 minutes until the top is browned and slightly puffed.

Cheesy chicken pasta with broccoli

For a vegetarian version, double the amount of broccoli and use vegetable instead of chicken broth.

8 ounces pasta shapes, e.g. fusilli
1 cup broccoli florets
2 tablespoons butter
1 large shallot, or 2 small, chopped
1 garlic clove, crushed
3 tablespoons all-purpose flour
1 cup milk
1¼ cups chicken broth
¾ cup grated sharp Cheddar cheese
⅓ cup grated Parmesan cheese
1 cooked chicken breast, shredded
   (about 4 ounces/1½ cups)
Salt and pepper
Sweet smoked Spanish paprika
   (optional)

◉ Cook the pasta following the package directions, adding the broccoli for the last 3 minutes.

◉ While the pasta is cooking, melt the butter in a large saucepan and sauté the shallot and garlic for 2 to 3 minutes, until softened. Add the flour and stir to make a paste, then whisk in the milk and broth to make a smooth sauce; you may find it easier to do this off the heat.

◉ Bring the sauce to a boil, stirring constantly, then remove from the heat and stir in the cheeses and chicken.

◉ Drain the pasta and broccoli and return to the pan. Add the sauce and toss to coat, then season to taste. Sweet smoked Spanish paprika, if using, adds a delicious flavor to this dish.

Spanish paprika chicken pasta

The paprika adds a nice smoky flavor to this dish.

2 teaspoons olive oil
1 small red onion, finely chopped
½ red bell pepper, diced
1 garlic clove, crushed
½ teaspoon smoked Spanish
   paprika
1 chicken breast, sliced into
   small pieces
¼ cup coarsely chopped chorizo
1 (14-ounce) can diced tomatoes
½ teaspoon tomato paste
½ teaspoon finely chopped fresh
   thyme leaves
6 ounces pasta shells
3 ounces fresh mozzarella, cubed

◉ Heat the oil in a saucepan on low heat. Add the onion, bell pepper, and garlic and fry gently for 5 minutes. Then add the paprika and chicken and fry for 1 minute.

◉ Mix in the chorizo, then the tomatoes, tomato paste, and thyme. Bring to a boil, then simmer for 5 minutes.

◉ Meanwhile, cook the pasta following the package directions, drain, then add to the sauce. Mix and add the mozzarella.

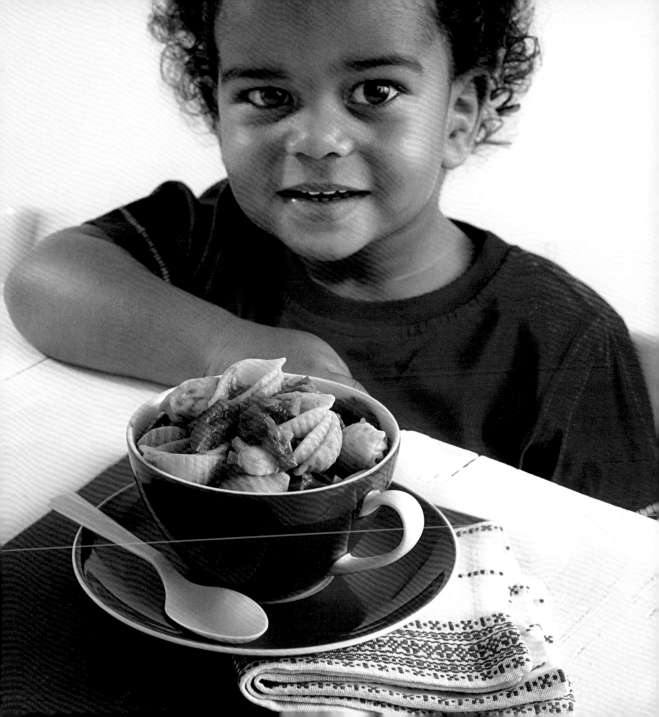

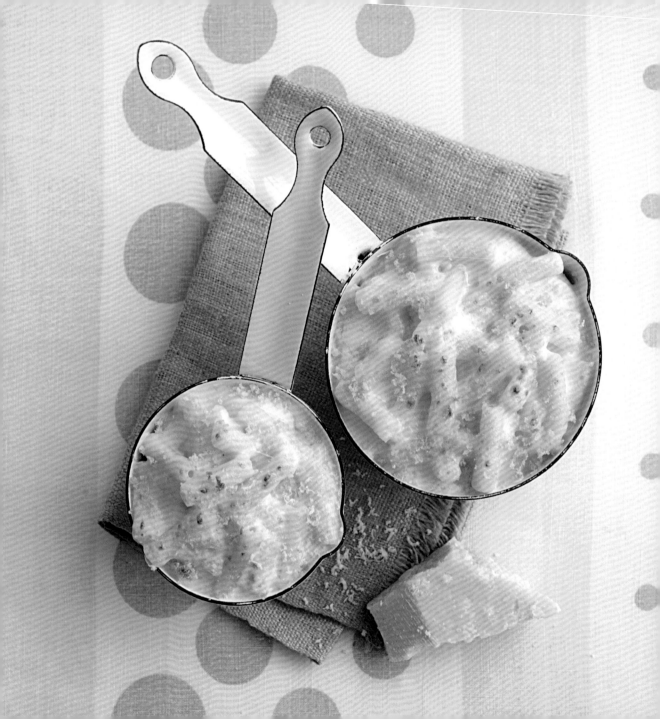

Macaroni and cheese

This is a delicious macaroni, made with three cheeses.

SUITABLE FOR FREEZING
MAKES 8 PORTIONS
6 ounces macaroni
2½ cups milk
3 tablespoons cornstarch
¾ cup grated sharp Cheddar cheese
¾ cup grated Gruyère cheese
⅔ cup grated Parmesan cheese
½ cup mascarpone
¼ teaspoon Dijon mustard
Salt and pepper

For the topping
⅓ cup bread crumbs (1 slice bread)
¼ cup grated Parmesan cheese

◉ Cook the macaroni following the package directions. Drain and rinse under cold water. Heat 2 cups of milk until just boiling.

◉ Mix the cornstarch and the remaining ½ cup milk and whisk into the hot milk. Cook, whisking constantly, until the sauce thickens and comes to a boil.

◉ Whisk in the cheeses until melted, then the mascarpone and mustard. Stir in the pasta and season to taste. Transfer to a baking dish. Mix the bread crumbs and Parmesan and sprinkle on top. Broil until golden.

Spaghetti carbonara

Carbonara is a perennial favorite with kids of all ages.

NOT SUITABLE FOR FREEZING
MAKES 4 PORTIONS
8 ounces spaghetti
½ tablespoon olive oil
1 cup diced pancetta
½ cup heavy cream
2 egg yolks
½ cup grated Parmesan cheese
Salt and freshly ground black pepper

◉ Cook the spaghetti in lightly salted boiling water until al dente.

◉ Heat the oil in a frying pan and sauté the pancetta for 3 to 4 minutes, until browned.

◉ In a bowl, whisk the cream, egg yolks, Parmesan, salt, and pepper. Drain the pasta and return to the saucepan. Immediately stir in the egg and cheese mixture until well combined. Add the pancetta, toss with the sauce, and gently heat through. You can thin the sauce with a little extra cream if necessary. Serve immediately with some Parmesan.

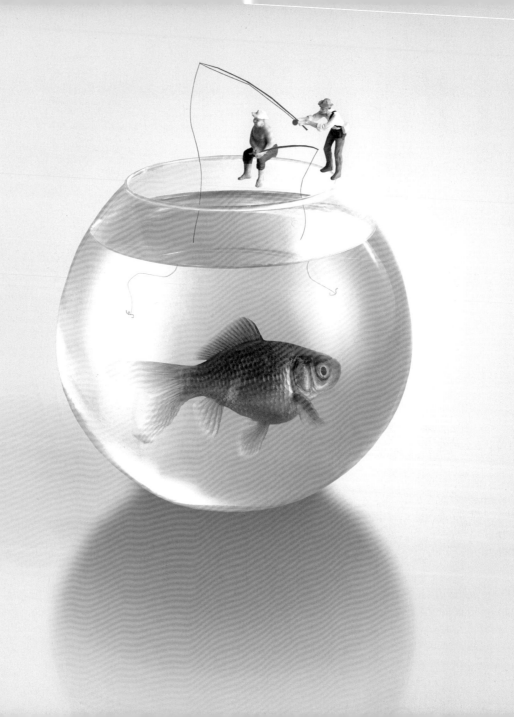

Fast fish

Homemade fish sticks

You can halve the quantities to make four portions.

1¼ cups fresh bread crumbs (made
　from 3 slices whole-grain bread,
　crusts removed)
½ cup grated Parmesan cheese
1 tablespoon chopped fresh chives
⅓ cup all-purpose flour for dusting
1 egg
1 tablespoon cold water
Pinch of salt
2 large flounder fillets, skin removed,
　cut into 8 small pieces
2 tablespoons canola oil for frying

◉ Put the bread crumbs, cheese, and chives in a food processor and whiz to combine. Spread the bread crumb mixture on one plate and the flour on a second plate. Beat the egg with the water and salt in a shallow dish.

◉ Dust the fish fillets with the flour, then dip in egg, and coat in bread crumbs. Lay the fillets on a cutting board or baking sheet.

◉ Heat the oil in a large frying pan. Fry the fillets for 2 minutes, each side, until golden and cooked through. You will probably need to do this in two to three batches. Blot with paper towels before serving.

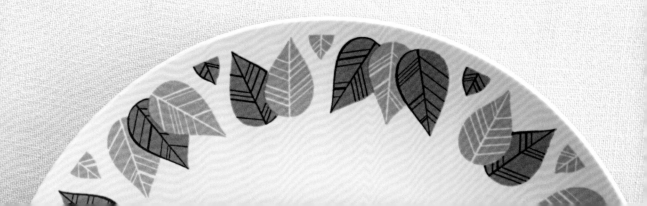

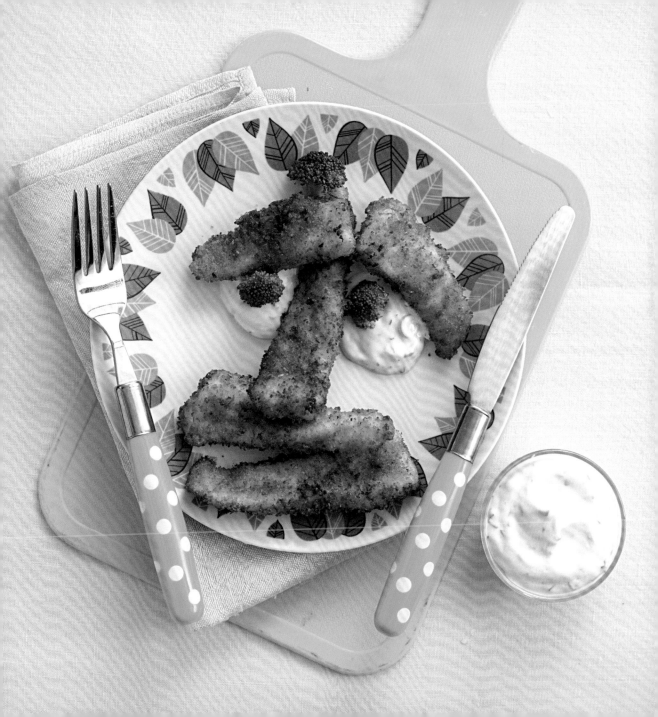

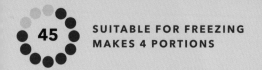

SUITABLE FOR FREEZING
MAKES 4 PORTIONS

Shrimp laksa

The coconut milk makes this a smooth-tasting curry that will go down a treat.

1 small onion, thinly sliced
1 tablespoon canola oil
½ teaspoon grated fresh ginger
2 tablespoons korma curry paste,
 or 1 tablespoon curry powder
1 (14-ounce) can coconut milk
1 cup chicken, fish, or
 vegetable broth
2 teaspoons soy sauce
1 teaspoon fish sauce
1 teaspoon honey
1 large carrot, julienned
8 ounces raw shrimp, heads
 and shells removed
1 cup frozen peas
4 ounces dry rice vermicelli,
 prepared following the package
 directions

Optional garnishes
Scallions, thinly sliced
Cilantro leaves
Chopped chiles
Lime wedges

◉ Sauté the onion in the oil for 5 minutes, until soft. Add the ginger and curry paste and cook for 1 minute. Then add the coconut milk, broth, soy sauce, fish sauce, and honey.

◉ Bring to a boil, then reduce the heat, add the carrot and simmer for 5 minutes.

◉ Add the shrimp and simmer for 2 to 3 minutes, until the shrimp turns pink. Then add the peas and cook for 1 to 2 minutes, until the peas have warmed through. Stir in the rice vermicelli and ladle into bowls. If you wish, garnish with one of the suggested options.

Tagliatelle with tomato and tuna

I've put olives as optional here as they can be an acquired taste, but I've found many young children really like olives.

1 tablespoon olive oil
⅓ cup diced red onion
¼ cup diced red bell pepper
¼ cup peeled and grated apple
1 (14-ounce) can diced tomatoes
¼ cup tomato paste
1 teaspoon sugar
¾ cup vegetable broth
7 ounces tagliatelle
Salt and pepper
1 (12-ounce) can tuna in water, drained
¾ cup grated sharp Cheddar cheese
Black olives (optional)

◉ Heat the oil in a large, deep frying pan and sauté the onion for 3 minutes, until translucent. Add the bell pepper and cook for 5 to 6 minutes, until the vegetables are soft. Add the apple, tomatoes, tomato paste, sugar, and broth and bring to a boil, then simmer for 30 minutes, until thickened.

◉ Blend the sauce until smooth, then return to the pan.

◉ Meanwhile, cook the pasta following the package directions, drain, and toss with the sauce. Season with salt and pepper.

◉ Flake the tuna and fold into the pasta.

◉ Transfer to a baking dish and sprinkle with the cheese. Grill until the cheese has melted and is bubbling.

◉ Add a handful of black olives to the tomato sauce, if you like.

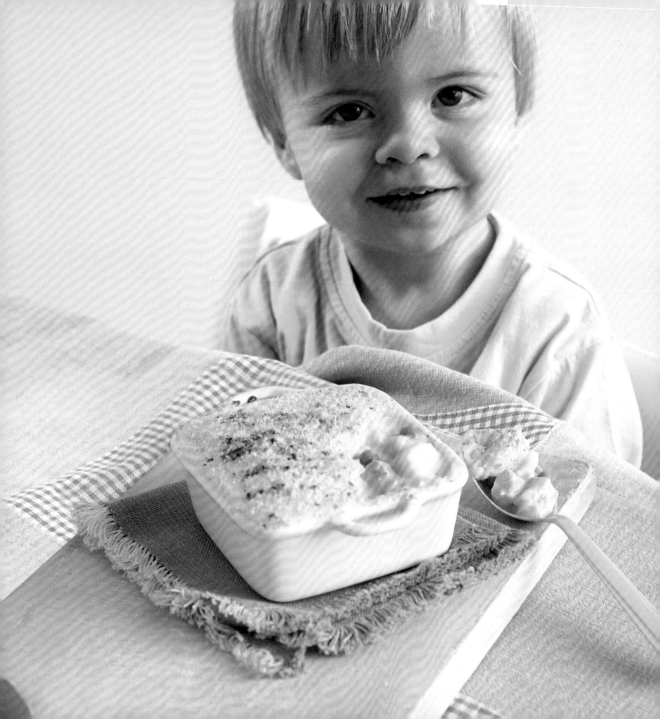

Little fish pies with peas

These little fish pies are a great warming dish, and very nutritious.

14 ounces Yukon Gold potatoes, peeled and cubed
2 tablespoons butter
2 shallots, finely diced
1½ teaspoons rice wine vinegar
3 tablespoons all-purpose flour
1½ cups milk
½ cup grated Parmesan cheese
½ teaspoon lemon juice
Salt and pepper
4 ounces salmon fillet, skin removed, cubed
4 ounces cod fillet, skin removed, cubed
⅓ cup cooked peas
Paprika

◉ Preheat the oven to 350°F.

◉ For the mashed potatoes, put the potatoes into cold water. Bring to a boil and simmer for 10 to 12 minutes, until tender. Drain well, then mash.

◉ Melt the butter in a saucepan. Add the shallots and sauté for 5 to 8 minutes, until soft. Add the vinegar and sauté until most of the vinegar has evaporated. Add the flour and mix to form a roux. Blend in 1¼ cups of the milk. Stir over gentle heat until thickened.

◉ Remove from the heat and stir in 5 tablespoons of the Parmesan and the lemon juice. Season and add the fish. Stir in the peas, then spoon into the bases of four (4-inch) diameter ramekins.

◉ Put the pan of mashed potatoes back onto the heat. Add the remaining ¼ cup milk and season to taste. Stir until hot, then spoon on top of the fish mixture and use the tines of a fork to make a pattern on the surface.

◉ Sprinkle with the remaining Parmesan and a little paprika. Place on a baking sheet.

◉ Bake for 15 to 20 minutes until lightly browned on top and bubbling at the edges.

Fusilli with salmon and shrimp

25

A simple, light fish dish.

NOT SUITABLE FOR FREEZING
MAKES 4 PORTIONS
8 ounces fusilli pasta
7 tablespoons fish broth
1 cup crème fraîche or heavy cream
Juice of ½ lemon (about 2 tablespoons)
2 tablespoons chopped fresh dill plus extra for garnish
6 ounces cooked shrimp
6 ounces cooked salmon
1 to 2 tomatoes, peeled and diced (optional)
Salt and pepper

◉ Cook the pasta following the package directions. Reserve one cup of the pasta cooking water, then drain the pasta and set aside.

◉ Put the broth in a saucepan and boil until reduced by half. Reduce the heat to low, stir in the crème fraîche, lemon juice, and dill. Add the shrimp and salmon and warm through, then add the pasta and carefully toss together, adding a splash of the reserved pasta water if the sauce gets too thick.

◉ Stir in the tomatoes, if using. Season with a little salt and pepper and serve immediately, sprinkle with extra dill.

Salmon with Parmesan crust and tomato salsa

25

The salsa adds a nice juiciness to this recipe.

NOT SUITABLE FOR FREEZING
MAKES 4 PORTIONS
1 cup fresh white bread crumbs
2 tablespoons grated Parmesan cheese
1 tablespoon finely chopped chives
½ cup all-purpose flour
1 pound middle-cut salmon, skin removed
1 egg, beaten
2 tablespoon olive oil

For the salsa
3 large tomatoes, seeded and coarsely chopped
2 tablespoons chopped fresh basil
3 scallions, thinly sliced
1 tablespoon olive oil
1 tablespoon rice wine vinegar
Pinch of sugar (optional)

◉ Mix the bread crumbs, cheese, and chives. Spread on a plate. Put the flour on another plate.

◉ Slice the salmon into eight pieces. Toss each piece in the flour, then the egg, and coat in the bread crumbs. Heat the oil in a frying pan over medium heat. Fry the salmon for 3 to 4 minutes on each side, until golden, crispy, and cooked through.

To make the salsa
Put all the ingredients into a mixing bowl and toss together. Serve with the salmon.

Sweet chili salmon and simple stir-fry noodles

Children may prefer to have the salmon broken into large flakes or cut into cubes and tossed with the noodles.

For the noodles
1 tablespoon canola oil
1 small onion, thinly sliced
½ teaspoon grated fresh ginger
1 garlic clove, crushed
1¼ cups bean sprouts, or
  4 ounces of your favorite
  stir-fry vegetable mixture
4 ounces dry Chinese (chow mein)
  noodles, prepared following the
  package directions
1 tablespoon soy sauce
1 tablespoon Asian sesame oil

For the salmon
2 tablespoons sweet chili sauce
1 teaspoon rice wine vinegar
1 teaspoon honey
1 teaspoon soy sauce
½ teaspoon grated fresh ginger
2 (4-ounce) salmon fillets

⦿ Heat the oil in a wok and stir-fry the onion for 4 to 5 minutes, until soft and slightly browned. Add the ginger and garlic and fry for 1 minute, then add the bean sprouts or stir-fry vegetables and cook for 2 minutes, until the vegetables start to soften.

⦿ Add the noodles and cook for 1 to 2 minutes to reheat, then stir in the soy sauce and sesame oil and set aside.

⦿ Preheat the broiler to high and line the broiler pan with foil. Mix the sweet chili sauce, vinegar, honey, soy sauce, and ginger.

⦿ Broil the skin side of the salmon for 2 minutes, then turn over and spoon 1 teaspoon of the sweet chili glaze on top of each piece of salmon, spreading it out and down the sides slightly.

⦿ Broil for 2 minutes, spread another teaspoon of glaze on each salmon and broil for 3 to 6 minutes more, until the salmon is cooked through and the top is glazed and slightly caramelized at the edges.

⦿ Add the leftover glaze to the noodles and stir-fry over high heat for about 2 minutes until piping hot. Serve with the salmon.

Bag-baked trout with ginger soy

Trout is an oily fish, so it's a good source of omega-3. It has a milder flavor than salmon, so it's a good fish to try, as children may find salmon a little overpowering. Baking fish in foil or parchment paper seals in all the nutrients and flavor.

Canola oil for greasing
1 small rainbow trout, filleted
    and bones removed
6 thin slices fresh ginger
1 teaspoon soy sauce
1 teaspoon rice wine vinegar
1 tablespoon water

For the dressing
1 tablespoon canola oil
2 scallions, finely chopped
½ teaspoon grated fresh ginger
1 teaspoon soy sauce
1 teaspoon rice wine vinegar
½ teaspoon Asian sesame oil
½ teaspoon honey

● ● ● ● ● ● ● ● ● ● ● ● ● ●
PIN BONES
Filleted trout will often have pin bones that must be removed for children. This is very easy to do. Run your finger down the flesh side of the fillet; you will feel the pin bones. You can easily pluck them out using a pair of tweezers.

◉ Preheat the oven to 400°F, with a baking sheet in the oven.

◉ Cut two large pieces of foil or parchment paper and grease with canola oil. Lay the fish fillets on the foil or parchment paper and place 3 slices of ginger on each one.

◉ Mix the soy sauce, vinegar, and water and spoon over the fish. Wrap the foil or parchment paper to form a parcel, scrunching the foil or using metal paper clips to help secure the parchment paper. Put on the baking sheet and bake for 10 minutes.

◉ Meanwhile, heat the canola oil in a small frying pan. Add the scallions and ginger and when they start to sizzle, take the frying pan off the heat and set aside.

◉ Unwrap the fish and remove the ginger. Transfer the fish to plates, using a spatula and sliding it between the fish and the skin to remove the skin from the cooked fish.

◉ Pour any juices left in the foil or parchment paper into the frying pan, then add the soy sauce, vinegar, sesame oil, and honey. Stir together, then spoon over the fish, and serve immediately.

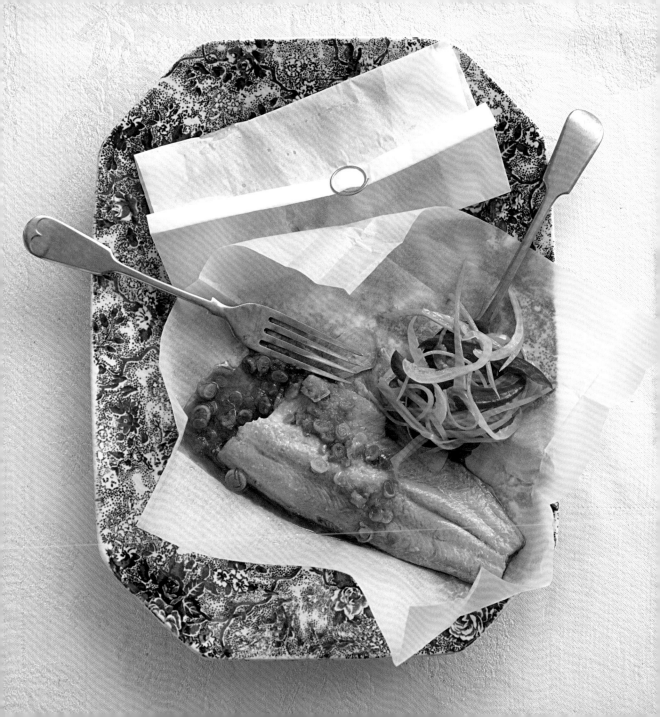

Asian rice salad with shrimp

 20

NOT SUITABLE FOR FREEZING
MAKES 3 PORTIONS
½ cup Thai jasmine rice
¼ red bell pepper, diced
3 tablespoons drained canned corn
2 scallions, thinly sliced
4 ounces small cooked shrimp
Cilantro leaves for garnish

For the dressing
2 tablespoons rice wine vinegar
2 teaspoons sugar
1 teaspoon mirin
1 teaspoon canola oil

◉ Cook the rice following the package directions. Drain, rinse with cold water, and leave to drain in a colander for 10 minutes. Then transfer to a bowl.

◉ Stir in the bell pepper, corn, scallions, and shrimp.

◉ Whisk the dressing ingredients. Pour over the salad and stir to combine.

◉ Cover and chill. Serve decorated with cilantro leaves.

Asian cod balls with plum dipping sauce

25

SUITABLE FOR FREEZING
MAKES ABOUT 20 BALLS
8 ounces cod fillet, skin removed
1 bunch scallions, finely chopped
1½ tablespoons sweet chili sauce
¼ cup grated Parmesan cheese
1 teaspoon soy sauce
1 egg yolk
½ cup panko bread crumbs
2 tablespoons canola oil

For the sauce
3 tablespoons plum sauce
2 tablespoons water
2 teaspoons soy sauce

◉ Whiz the cod in a food processor until coarsely chopped, then transfer to a bowl.

◉ Add the scallions, chili sauce, cheese, soy sauce, egg yolk, and bread crumbs and mix together. Shape into 20 balls.

◉ Heat the oil in a frying pan. Fry the balls for 8 to 10 minutes, until lightly golden and cooked through.

To make the sauce
◉ Put all the ingredients into a small saucepan. Gently warm through and serve with the balls.

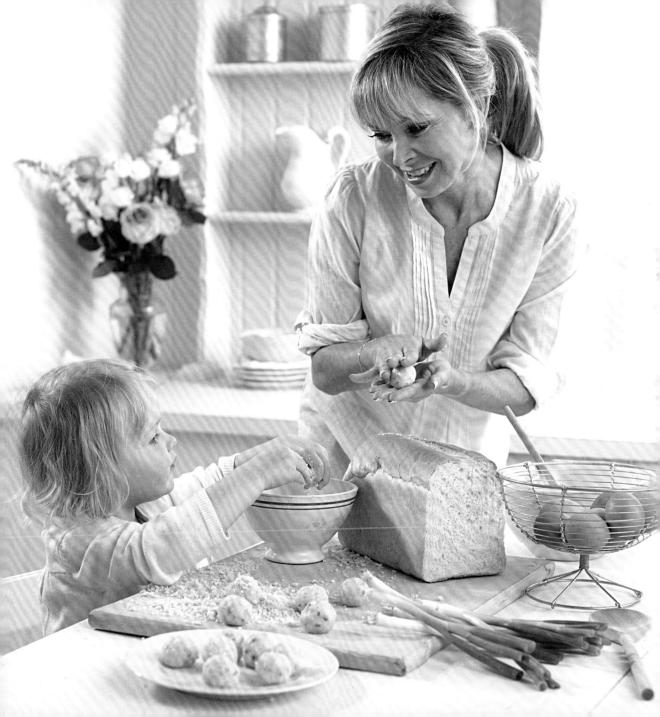

Mild korma curry with shrimp

Curry is one of my children's favorite meals, and this is a mild and fruity version. Serve with papadums and rice.

2 tablespoons olive oil
1 small onion, finely chopped
1 teaspoon grated fresh ginger
1 tablespoon korma or mild curry
    paste
1 teaspoon garam masala
1 cup canned diced tomatoes
1 cup coconut milk
½ teaspoon lemon juice
½ to 1 teaspoon mango chutney
Salt and pepper
8 ounces shell-off raw jumbo shrimp

◉ Heat the oil in a saucepan. Add the onion and sauté for 3 minutes. Add the ginger, curry paste, and garam masala and fry for 2 minutes.

◉ Add the tomatoes, coconut milk, lemon juice, and mango chutney. Bring to a boil, then simmer, uncovered, for 8 to 10 minutes, stirring until it has reduced and is an orange-red color.

◉ Season and add the shrimp and cook for another 5 minutes, until they have turned pink and are cooked through.

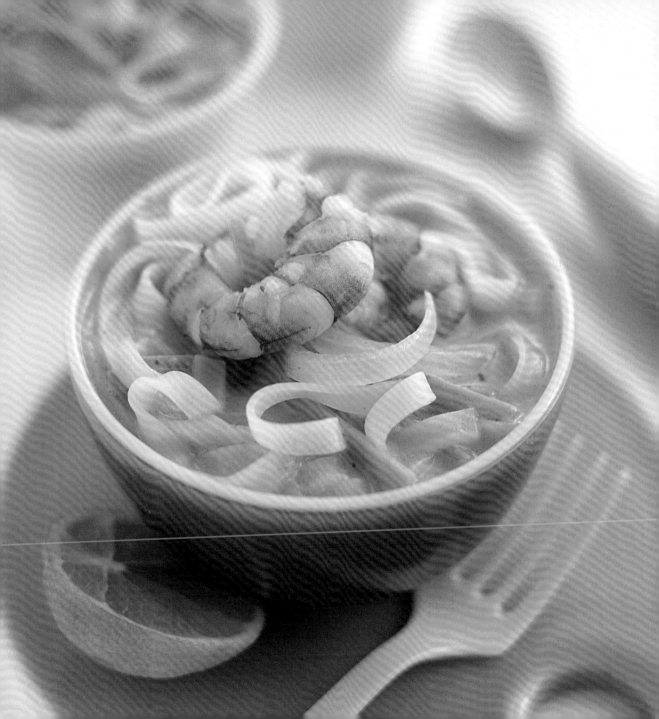

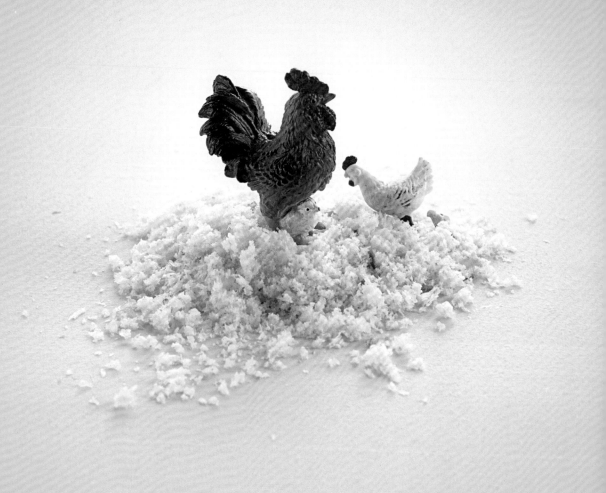

Express chicken and poultry

Quick sauces for chicken

Serve these sauces with grilled or panfried chicken.

Grilled chicken

NOT SUITABLE FOR FREEZING
MAKES 2 PORTIONS
2 boneless, skinless chicken breasts
1 tablespoon olive oil
1 garlic clove, peeled
Salt and pepper

◉ Cover the chicken breast fillets with plastic wrap and pound with a mallet to flatten them.

◉ Brush the fillets with oil and then run a cut garlic clove over them. Season with a little salt and pepper.

◉ Brush a grill pan with oil and when it is very hot cook the chicken on one side for 2 to 3 minutes. Reduce the heat and cook for another 3 minutes. Turn the chicken over and repeat.

◉ Cut the chicken into strips and serve with the tasty dipping sauces.

SAUCES
Mild curry

2 tablespoons mayonnaise
2 tablespoons Greek yogurt
1½ teaspoons mild korma curry paste
1 teaspoon honey
2 to 3 drops lemon juice

Easy barbecue

3 tablespoons ketchup
1 tablespoon honey
¼ teaspoon soy sauce
¼ teaspoon lemon juice
2 teaspoons water

Spicy tomato

3 tablespoons ketchup
1 tablespoon sweet chili sauce
1 tablespoon water
¼ teaspoon soy sauce

◉ Mix the ingredients for your dip of choice and serve with the cooked chicken or with vegetable sticks.

Chicken Bolognese

If your child is a fussy eater and picks out the vegetables, cook them until they are soft, add the tomatoes, and blend until smooth. Brown the chicken in a separate frying pan and add the remaining ingredients before simmering as per the recipe.

1 tablespoon olive oil
1 small onion, finely chopped
¼ red bell pepper, diced
1 medium carrot, diced
½ small celery stalk, diced (optional)
1 garlic clove, crushed
¼ teaspoon chopped fresh thyme
    leaves
8 ounces ground chicken
1 (14-ounce) can diced tomatoes
⅔ cup chicken broth
2 tablespoons tomato paste
1 tablespoon ketchup
1½ teaspoons sugar
Salt and pepper

◉ Heat the oil in a large saucepan over medium heat. Sauté the vegetables for 8 to 10 minutes, until soft. Add the garlic and thyme and cook for 1 minute.

◉ Add the chicken and turn up the heat slightly, then cook for 2 to 4 minutes, stirring and breaking up the chicken with a wooden spoon, until the chicken has browned slightly.

◉ Add the remaining ingredients, bring to a boil, then reduce the heat and simmer for 20 to 30 minutes until thickened. Season with salt and pepper.

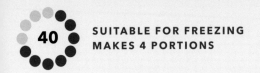
Little chicken and leek pies

Little ones will love to have mini portions in individual ramekin dishes. You can also prepare several at a time and freeze extra portions for days when you don't have time to cook.

1⅔ cups peeled and diced potatoes
1⅔ cups diced carrots
1 tablespoon butter
2 small leeks, coarsely chopped
8 ounces chicken tenders, cut into
    ¾ inch-cubes
3 mushrooms, sliced
2 tablespoons all-purpose flour
¾ cup milk
½ cup grated Cheddar cheese
2 tablespoons corn kernels
Salt and pepper

◉ Preheat the broiler.

◉ Put the potatoes and carrots into a saucepan. Bring to a boil and keep it there for 10 to 12 minutes, until soft. Drain, then mash until smooth.

◉ Melt the butter in a saucepan. Add the leeks and sauté for 5 minutes, until just soft. Add the chicken and fry for 2 minutes. Add the mushrooms and cook for 2 minutes. Sprinkle with the all-purpose flour. Blend in the milk and bring to a boil.

◉ Simmer for 5 minutes, until the chicken is cooked. Add three quarters of the cheese, the corn, and season with salt and pepper. Spoon into four ramekins (about 6 ounces). Spoon the mashed vegetables on top and sprinkle with the remaining cheese.

◉ Broil for 4 to 5 minutes, until lightly golden on top and bubbling around the edges.

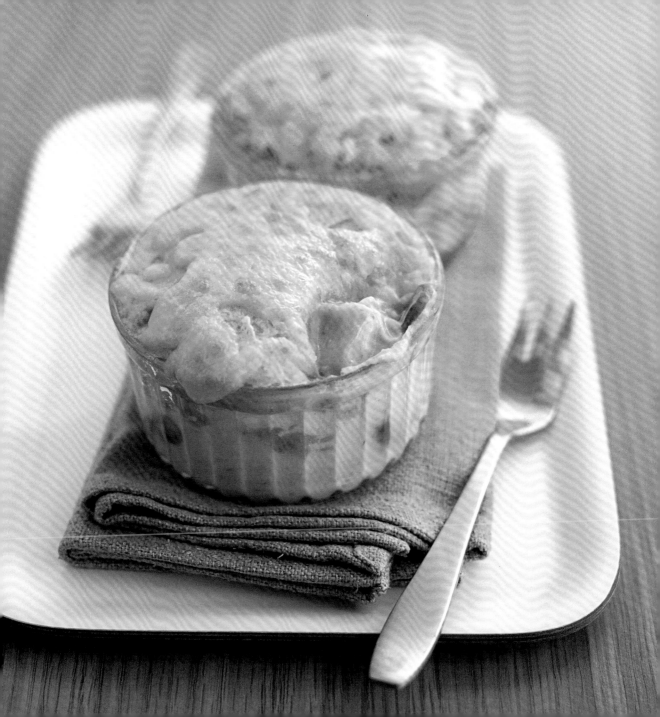

Chicken with ham and cheese

This recipe is a delicious way to stuff chicken breasts.

4 small boneless, skinless chicken
  breasts (about 4 ounces each)
¾ cup grated Gruyère cheese
4 small slices ham, finely chopped
4 tablespoons chopped chives
1 egg, beaten
1 cup fresh bread crumbs
Paprika
2 tablespoons oil

◉ Preheat the oven to 400°F.

◉ Put the chicken breasts on a cutting board. Cover with plastic wrap and, using a mallet, lightly pound the thicker part of the breast so that it is coarsely the same thickness.

◉ Carefully slice each breast three quarters of the way through the middle, still keeping one side attached. Mix the cheese, ham, and chives.

◉ Open one breast and put a quarter of the cheese mixture into the middle. Season and fold over the top. Push down so that it looks like a sandwich. Repeat with the remaining breasts.

◉ Brush each breast with egg wash. Carefully coat in bread crumbs. Sprinkle with paprika.

◉ Heat the oil in a large frying pan. Brown the chicken for 3 minutes on both sides, then place onto a baking sheet lined with parchment paper.

◉ Roast in the oven for 15 minutes until golden and cooked through. Leave for 3 minutes, then slice each breast into 3 to 4 slices to serve.

Chicken and gravy casserole

You could pound the chicken to flatten it and then marinate it in olive oil, garlic, and lemon (see page 84 for instructions on grilling).

2 teaspoons olive oil
Salt and pepper
2 ounces chicken tenders
2 small onions, thinly sliced
1 teaspoon finely chopped fresh
   thyme leaves
Pinch of brown sugar
1 teaspoon balsamic vinegar
1¼ cups beef broth
½ teaspoon Worcestershire sauce
¼ teaspoon tomato paste
2 teaspoons cornstarch

◉ Heat the oil in a deep frying pan. Season the chicken. Brown the chicken on both sides until lightly golden, then set aside on a plate.

◉ Add the onions to the pan. Sprinkle with the thyme. Cover and cook gently for 8 to 10 minutes, until very soft. Remove the lid, add the sugar and vinegar and fry until lightly golden.

◉ Add the broth, Worcestershire sauce, and tomato paste. Bring to a boil. Mix the cornstarch with a little cold water and add to the gravy. Stir until thickened.

◉ Return the chicken to the pan. Cover and simmer for 4 to 5 minutes, until cooked through. Serve with mashed potatoes.

Chicken meatballs in barbecue sauce

This is one of my children's favorite recipes. It's a good idea to make extra and put some child-size portions into the freezer so that they're there whenever you need them.

1 tablespoon olive oil
1 medium onion, finely chopped
1 garlic clove, crushed
7 tablespoons ketchup
1⅔ cups water
1½ tablespoons soy sauce
1 tablespoon brown sugar
2 teaspoons Worcestershire sauce
1 teaspoon balsamic vinegar
1 teaspoon lemon juice
1 tablespoon cornstarch

For the meatballs
1 slice white bread
2 skinless chicken breasts (about 8 ounces)
2 teaspoons chopped fresh thyme leaves
1 egg yolk
1 apple, peeled and grated

◉ Heat the oil in a saucepan over low heat. Add the onion and garlic and cook gently for 5 minutes, until soft.

◉ Divide the mixture in two and transfer half to a mixing bowl. Add the ketchup, water, soy sauce, brown sugar, Worcestershire sauce, and vinegar to the saucepan. Bring to a boil and simmer for 2 minutes.

◉ Add the lemon juice. Mix the cornstarch with a little cold water and add to the sauce, then stir until thickened.

To make the meatballs

◉ Whiz the slice of bread in a food processor to make bread crumbs. Transfer to the bowl with the cooked onion. Pulse the chicken in the food processor until it is finely chopped and add it to the onions and bread crumbs.

◉ Add the thyme, egg yolk, and apple to the bowl and gently mix. Shape into twenty-four balls.

◉ Heat a little oil in a frying pan. Fry the balls until lightly golden. Add to the sauce and simmer for 5 to 8 minutes, until cooked through.

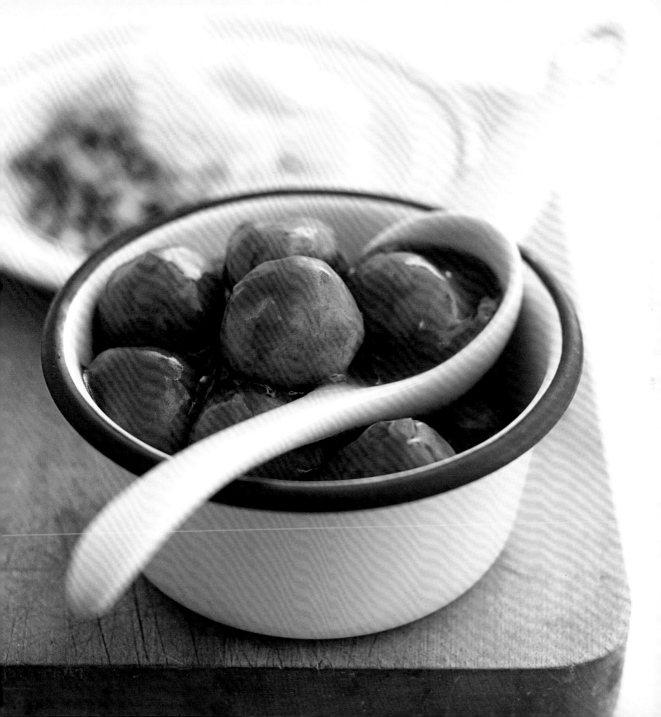

Toasted chicken tortilla

It's a nice idea to cook filled tortillas on a grill to make them crispy. They make great finger food.

6 ounces chicken tenders
1 teaspoon honey
Salt and pepper
2 tablespoons olive oil
3 scallions, thinly sliced
¼ cup grated Cheddar cheese
2 tablespoons coarsely chopped
   fresh basil
3 tablespoons corn kernels
¼ cup light mayonnaise
4 flour tortillas

◉ Put the chicken into a bowl. Drizzle with the honey and season with salt and pepper. Heat 1 tablespoon of the oil in a small frying pan and fry the chicken for 4 to 6 minutes until cooked, then set aside.

◉ Put the scallions, cheese, basil, corn, mayonnaise, and seasoning into a small bowl. Slice the chicken into small cubes, then add to the mixture and combine.

◉ Heat a grill pan until hot. Put the tortillas in the pan and gently warm through so that they are easier to roll. Place one on a work surface. Put a quarter of the mixture on one side of the tortilla, roll up, making sure that the end is underneath. Repeat with the remaining tortillas.

◉ Brush both sides with a little oil, then fry on both sides until char-grilled and the filling is warm and the cheese is starting to melt.

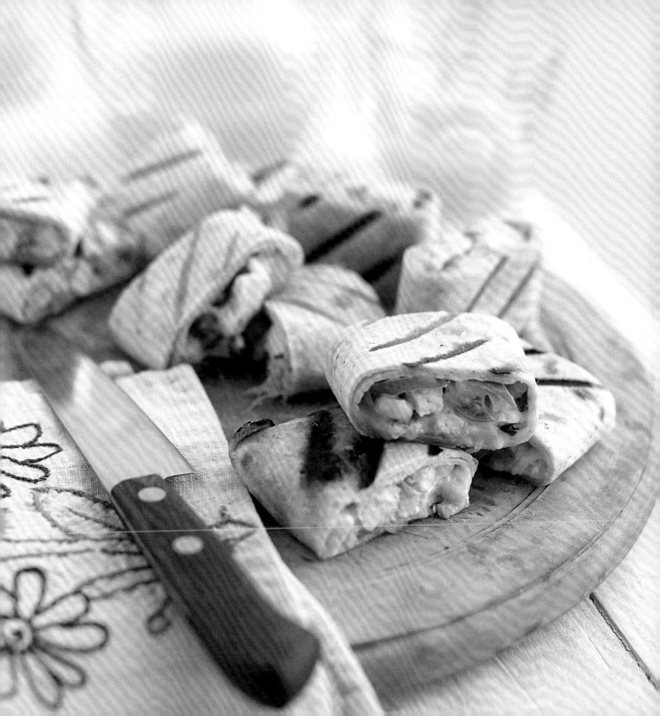

Marinated grilled chicken

Cut the marinated, grilled chicken into strips and serve with a selection of vegetables, depending on what your child likes.

For the marinade
1 tablespoon canola oil
1 teaspoon balsamic vinegar
2 teaspoons honey
1 teaspoon Asian sesame oil
1 teaspoon soy sauce

For the chicken
¼ small zucchini cut into 6 slices
¼ red bell pepper, cut in half
  lengthwise
¼ yellow bell pepper, cut in half
  lengthwise
1 large chicken breast

◉ Whisk the marinade ingredients in a bowl. Cut the chicken in half crosswise. Put the two slices on a cutting board, cover with plastic wrap and pound until about a ¼ inch thick. Transfer to a bowl. Put the vegetables in a separate bowl.

◉ Divide the marinade between the chicken and vegetables. Toss so that the chicken and vegetables are coated. Cover and marinate for 30 minutes (up to 1 hour).

◉ Heat a grill pan, brush with a little oil, and cook the zucchini for 1 to 1½ minutes on each side. Cook the bell peppers for 3 to 4 minutes on each side, and the chicken for 2 to 3 minutes on each side, or until the vegetables are soft and the chicken is cooked through.

◉ Transfer the marinade from the bowls to a saucepan. Bring to a boil and cook for 30 seconds, then spoon over the chicken and vegetables.

● ● ● ● ● ● ● ● ● ● ● ● ● ● ●
TIP
Do not serve the marinade without boiling first.

Tasty baked chicken

You can also make this recipe using chicken drumsticks, just remove some of the skin and trim away any excess fat. I have given the ingredients for two different glazes. Each glaze is enough for four chicken thighs.

For the mango chutney glaze
¼ cup mango chutney
1 tablespoon rice wine vinegar
    or lemon juice
1 tablespoon ketchup
Pinch of salt

For the sticky soy and ginger glaze
¼ cup honey
2 tablespoons soy sauce
1 tablespoon rice wine vinegar
1 garlic clove, crushed
1 teaspoon grated fresh ginger
1 tablespoon canola oil
4 skinless, bone-in chicken thighs

◉ Preheat the oven to 400°F.

◉ Whisk the glaze ingredients together. Put the chicken in an ovenproof baking dish or pan and score the flesh of each thigh two times.

◉ Season with pepper, then spoon on your chosen glaze. Cover with foil and bake for 15 minutes.

◉ Uncover, baste with the pan juices, and bake for 15 to 20 minutes more (if possible, baste again after 10 minutes), until the chicken is cooked through and the pan juices are sticky.

◉ Transfer the chicken to a plate and spoon the pan juices on top. Cool slightly before serving with rice, or baked potatoes, and green salad.

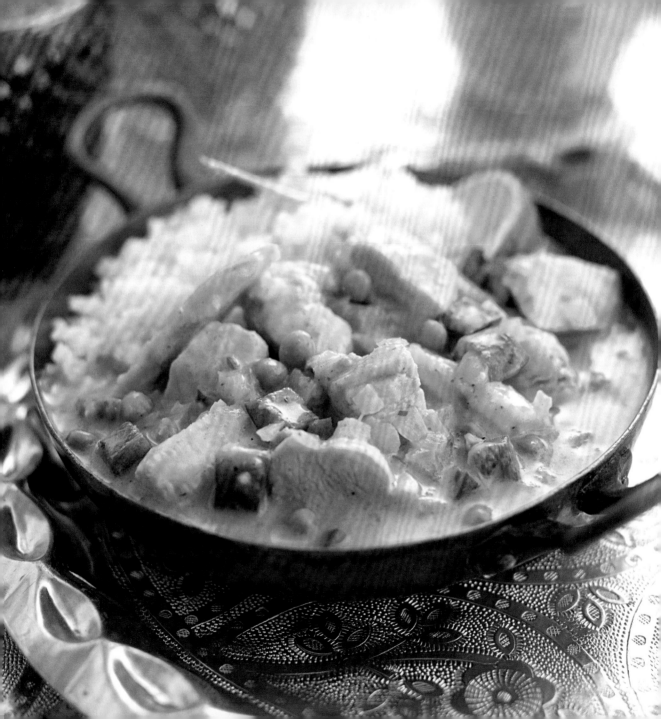

Fruity chicken korma

This is a delicious, mild, fruity curry.

1½ tablespoons canola oil
1 medium onion, finely chopped
½ red bell pepper, diced
1 small to medium apple, peeled, cored, and thinly sliced
2 skinless chicken breasts, diced
1½ tablespoons korma curry paste
1 teaspoon garam masala
½ cup low-fat coconut milk
½ cup chicken broth
1 to 1½ tablespoons mango chutney
1 tablespoon soy sauce
⅓ cup frozen corn kernels
½ cup frozen peas
2 teaspoons lime juice
1 teaspoon cornstarch
2 tablespoons cold water

◉ Heat the oil in a deep frying pan or wok.

◉ Add the onion and bell pepper and stir-fry for 3 minutes. Add the apple and sauté for 2 minutes. Add the chicken and stir-fry until browned. Add the curry paste and garam masala, then the coconut milk, broth, mango chutney, and soy sauce.

◉ Bring to a boil and simmer for 3 minutes. Add the corn, peas, and lime juice and cook for 2 to 3 minutes. Mix the cornstarch with the water. Add to the curry and stir until slightly thickened. Serve with rice.

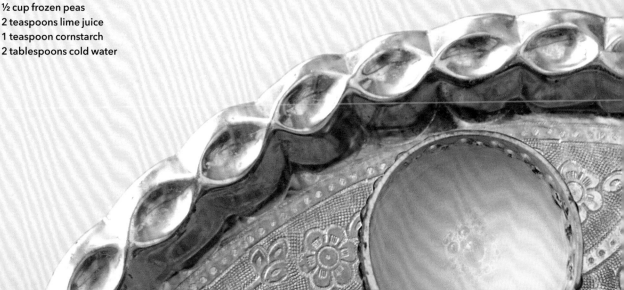

Tasty chicken and rice

This is great for lunch boxes or a light meal; the honey–soy sauce dressing is delicious. For speed you can buy parboiled rice that is ready in ten minutes.

⅔ cup long-grain rice
1 carrot, peeled and finely diced
6 scallions, thinly sliced
3 ounces cherry tomatoes,
    quartered
¼ cup drained canned corn
1 cooked chicken breast, diced
Salt and pepper

Dressing
1 teaspoon honey
1½ tablespoons soy sauce
1½ tablespoons rice wine vinegar
1½ tablespoons Asian sesame oil
2 tablespoons olive oil

◉ Cook the rice in boiling water following the package directions, drain, and let cool.

◉ Add the carrot, scallions, tomatoes, corn, and chicken and season with salt and pepper.

◉ Mix the honey, soy sauce, vinegar, sesame oil, and olive oil. Pour over the rice and serve.

Honey and soy-glazed drumsticks

You can marinate the chicken overnight if you have the time.

1 teaspoon finely grated fresh
   ginger
2 teaspoons soy sauce
1 teaspoon honey
1 teaspoon olive oil
4 small chicken drumsticks
Salt and pepper

◉ Preheat the oven to 400°F. Put the ginger, soy sauce, honey, and oil into a bowl. Mix well. Line a baking sheet with foil or parchment paper.

◉ It is important to score the drumsticks before you marinate them so that they cook all the way through. Put the drumsticks into the marinade. Toss to coat and season with salt and pepper. Pour onto the baking sheet. Roast for 20 to 30 minutes, turning halfway through. Remove from the baking sheet, wrap the ends in foil, and serve.

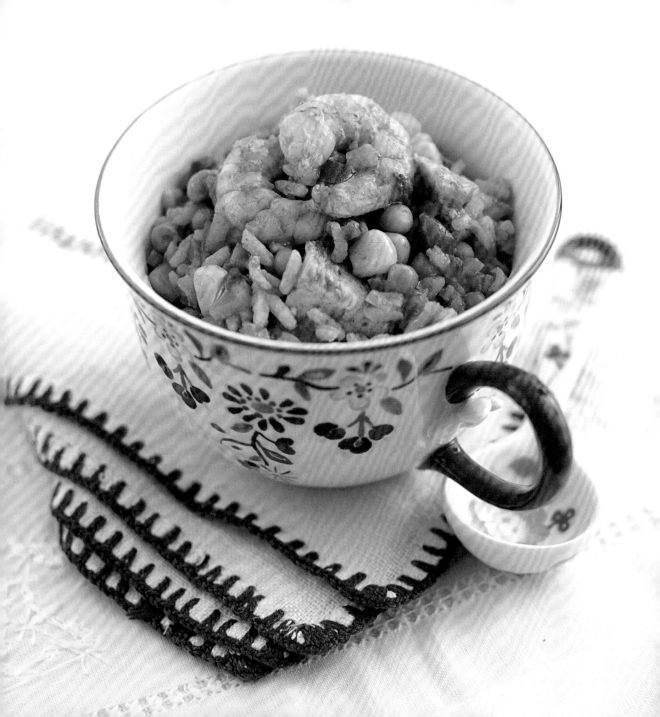

Jambalaya

The beauty of this dish is that you can substitute or add any ingredients you wish, so it's a great way of using up leftovers. If you like spicy food sauté ½ cup diced chorizo with the vegetables and remove the paprika.

1 tablespoon olive oil
1 medium onion, finely chopped
1 medium carrot, diced
¼ red bell pepper, diced
½ celery stalk, diced
1 garlic clove, crushed
¼ teaspoon chopped fresh thyme
   leaves
½ teaspoon paprika
1 cup basmati or long-grain rice
1 (14-ounce) can diced tomatoes
1 cup chicken broth
4 to 6 drops Tabasco, or to taste
1 cooked chicken breast (about
   4 ounces)
4 ounces cooked shrimp
⅔ cup frozen peas
1 cup drained canned corn
Salt and pepper

◉ Heat the oil in a large saucepan or wok with a lid.

◉ Sauté the onion, carrot, bell pepper, and celery for 8 to 10 minutes, until soft.

◉ Add the garlic, thyme, and paprika and cook for 1 minute. Add the rice, tomatoes, broth, and Tabasco and bring to a boil. Cover and simmer for 15 minutes, or until the rice is just tender.

◉ Uncover and add the chicken, shrimp, peas, and corn. Cover and cook for 5 minutes more, until everything is hot. Season with salt and pepper and stir with a fork. Serve with extra Tabasco, if you wish.

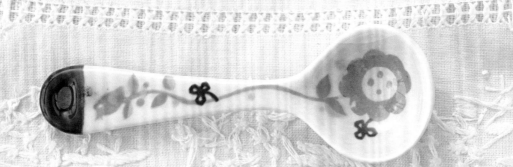

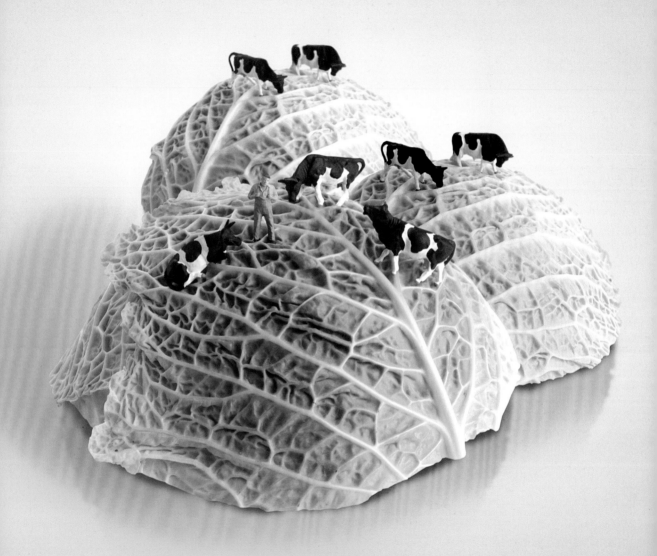

Meat in minutes

Cajun beef and onion wraps

These wraps make a tasty and filling snack or lunch.

2 teaspoons olive oil
8 ounces top loin steak, thinly sliced
1 teaspoon honey
1 small red onion, thinly sliced
1 red bell pepper, thinly sliced
1¼ cups sliced mushrooms
1 garlic clove, crushed
1½ teaspoons ground coriander
½ teaspoon sweet smoked paprika
1 teaspoon soy sauce
6 flour tortillas
½ cup grated Cheddar cheese
1 head Boston lettuce, shredded

◉ Heat the oil in a frying pan. Mix the steak with the honey and fry for 2 to 3 minutes, until browned. Transfer to a plate.

◉ Add the onion and pepper to the pan and fry for 5 minutes. Add the mushrooms and garlic and fry for another 2 minutes, then return the steak to the pan.

◉ Sprinkle with the coriander and paprika. Add the soy sauce and remove from the heat.

◉ Warm the tortillas in the microwave. Spoon some of the filling in the middle. Sprinkle with a little cheese and lettuce. Fold in the end of the tortilla and roll up.

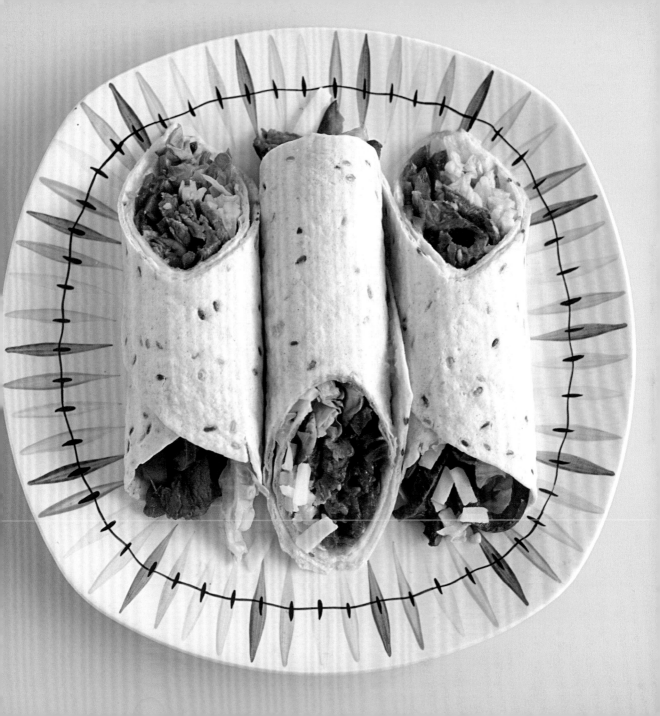

Barbecue beef Sloppy Joe

It's best to cook the beef for thirty minutes as it makes it more tender. You could also chop the beef in a food processor for a few seconds.

1 tablespoon olive oil
1 medium red onion, chopped
1 garlic clove, crushed
1 tablespoon balsamic vinegar
8 ounces lean ground beef
1 (14-ounce) can diced tomatoes
¼ cup ketchup
½ teaspoon Worcestershire sauce
½ teaspoon soy sauce
1 teaspoon light brown sugar
Salt and pepper

⦿ Heat the oil in a large frying pan with high sides, or a wok. Sauté the onion and garlic for 5 minutes, add the vinegar and the beef and cook for 2 minutes, stirring until the beef is browned, then add the remaining ingredients.

⦿ Bring to a boil, then reduce the heat and simmer for 25 to 30 minutes. Season to taste with salt and pepper. Add a splash of water if the sauce gets too dry. It should be slightly sloppy (hence the name).

To serve
⦿ Sloppy Joe is usually served on a split hamburger bun, but you could also serve it with rice. Cook ¾ cup rice following the package directions. Drain, spoon onto plates, and then top with the meat sauce.

Quick Bolognese

Always a favorite—and the recipe below is a quick and easy way to make Bolognese.

1 tablespoon olive oil
1 medium onion, chopped
1 garlic clove, crushed
1 medium carrot, grated
¼ red bell pepper, coarsely
   chopped
1 (14-ounce) can diced tomatoes
8 ounces lean ground beef
2 tablespoons tomato paste
1 teaspoon sugar
Salt and pepper
Parmesan cheese, grated (optional)

◉ Heat the oil in a large frying pan with high sides, or a wok, and sauté the onion and garlic for 5 minutes, until the onion is translucent.

◉ Meanwhile, whiz the carrot, bell pepper, and diced tomatoes to a puree in a food processor.

◉ Add the beef to the frying pan and cook for 2 minutes, until it is browned, then add the tomato mixture, tomato paste, and sugar. Bring to a boil, then simmer for 25 minutes, stirring occasionally. Add a splash of water if the sauce gets too dry. Season to taste with salt and pepper.

To serve with pasta
◉ While the sauce is simmering, bring a large saucepan of salted water to a boil, add 8 ounces of pasta and boil for the time specified on the package. Reserve a cupful of pasta cooking water before draining the pasta. Stir the cooked pasta into the sauce at the end of the cooking time, adding a little of the reserved pasta cooking water if the sauce gets too dry.

◉ Serve with grated Parmesan cheese.

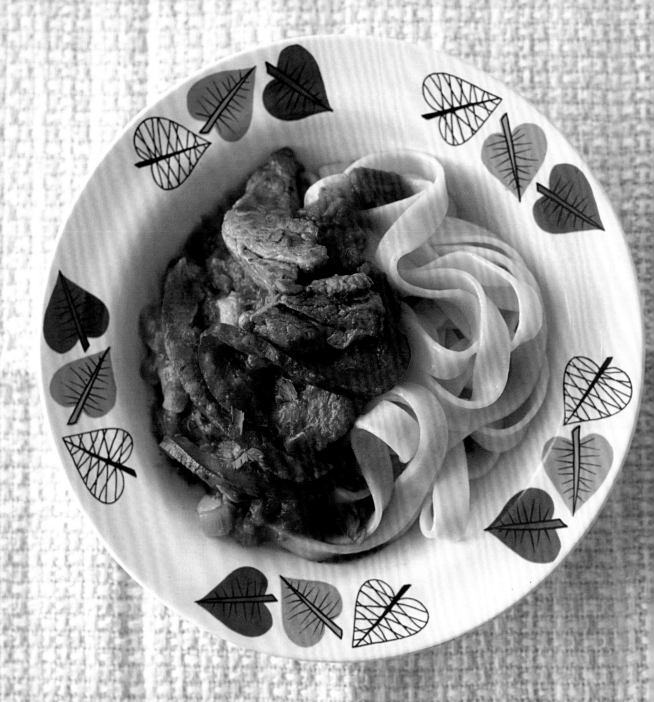

Annabel's goulash express

A delicious quick way to make a tasty goulash. Serve with noodles or rice.

12 ounces top loin steak,
   trimmed of fat
1 tablespoon olive oil
1 onion, chopped
1 garlic clove, crushed
½ red bell pepper, seeded and
   julienned
1 teaspoon sweet paprika
¼ teaspoon smoked paprika
1 (14-ounce) can diced tomatoes
2 tablespoons tomato paste
½ cup beef broth
½ teaspoon sugar
Salt and pepper
2 tablespoons crème fraîche or sour
   cream
1 tablespoon chopped fresh parsley
   (optional)

◉ Put the steak on a cutting board, cover with plastic wrap, and pound with a mallet or rolling pin until ⅛ inch thick. Cut into finger-size strips.

◉ Heat the oil in a wok or large frying pan. Sear the beef for 3 minutes; it should still be pink inside. Transfer the beef to a plate and set aside.

◉ Return the wok to the heat and add the onion, garlic, and bell pepper. Sauté for 2 minutes until soft, then add both of the paprikas and sauté for 3 minutes.

◉ Add the tomatoes, tomato paste, broth, and sugar, bring to a boil and simmer for 10 minutes. Turn the heat to very low, add the beef to the wok and cook for 5 minutes. Try not to boil the sauce once the beef has been added.

◉ Remove from the heat, season to taste with salt and pepper, and stir in the crème fraîche. Sprinkle with the parsley, if using.

To serve with the goulash
◉ Buttered noodles are a common accompaniment. Cook 8 ounces of tagliatelle following the package directions, drain, and toss with a pat of butter. Divide between 3 or 4 plates and spoon on the goulash.

◉ Alternatively cook ¾ cup of rice following the package directions, drain, and divide between 3 or 4 plates, then spoon on the goulash.

Mild massaman beef curry

Massaman curry comes from southern Thailand and is one of the few Thai curries made with beef.

12 ounces top loin steak, trimmed of fat
1 tablespoon canola oil
1 small onion, chopped
1 garlic clove, crushed
½ teaspoon ground coriander
½ teaspoon ground cumin
½ teaspoon grated fresh ginger
2 teaspoons red Thai curry paste, or to taste
8 small baby white potatoes (8 ounces), quartered
1 (14-ounce) can coconut milk
½ cup beef broth
1 teaspoon soy sauce
1 teaspoon sugar
2 teaspoons lime juice

Optional garnishes
1 tablespoon chopped fresh cilantro
1 tablespoon chopped peanuts
Wedge of lime
Snow peas, julienned

◉ Put the steak on a cutting board. Cover with a piece of plastic wrap and pound with a mallet or rolling pin until the steak is ⅛ inch thick. Cut into finger-size pieces.

◉ Heat the oil in a wok and sear the beef for 2 to 3 minutes. It should still be pink inside. Transfer to a plate and set aside.

◉ Return the wok to the heat and sauté the onion, garlic, coriander, and cumin for 5 minutes. Add the ginger, curry paste, potatoes, coconut milk, broth, soy sauce, and sugar. Bring to a boil and cook for 10 minutes, or until the potatoes are tender.

◉ Reduce the heat to low and add the beef. Cook for 5 minutes more. Try not to let the curry boil once the meat has been added. Stir in the lime juice. Taste after the first teaspoon has been added and add more if you like.

To serve the curry
◉ Traditionally the curry is served in bowls sprinkled with chopped cilantro and peanuts, with a wedge of lime to squeeze over it, and some papadums or naan bread.

◉ If you prefer to serve with rice, then omit the potatoes and just simmer the sauce for 10 minutes. Cook ¾ cup of rice following the package directions.

◉ Add a handful of snow peas, if using. Then add the beef to the curry for the last 5 minutes of cooking time. Drain the rice, divide between bowls, and spoon on the finished curry.

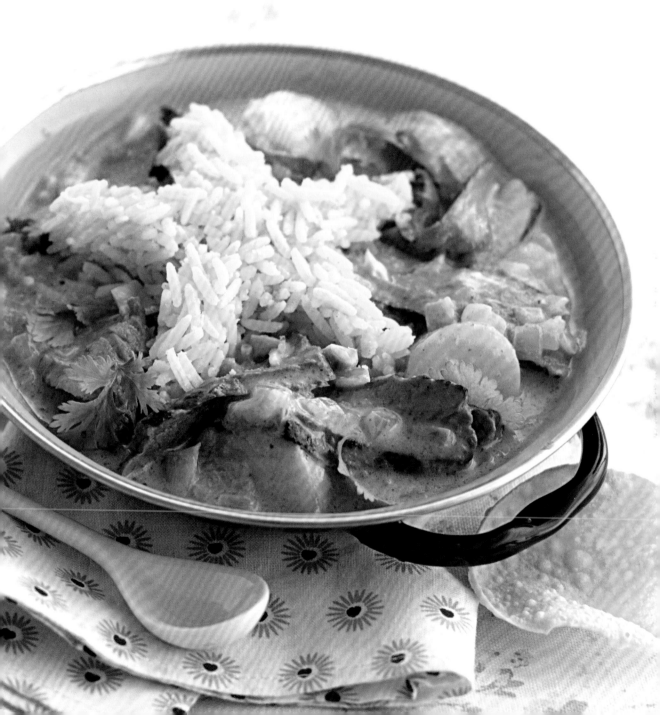

Thyme, garlic, and lemon lamb chops

These marinated lamb chops are beautifully tender.

4 sprigs fresh thyme
2 teaspoons lemon juice
1 garlic clove, crushed
2 tablespoons olive oil
4 frenched lamb rib chops

◉ Remove the leaves from the thyme sprigs and put in a bowl with the lemon juice, garlic, and oil. Add the chops and coat in the marinade. Marinate for as long as possible.

◉ Preheat the broiler to high. Put onto a baking sheet and broil about 8 inches away from the heat source for 8 to 10 minutes, turning over halfway through the cooking time. This makes a "pink" chop.

◉ Cook for 12 to 15 minutes for a well-done chop.

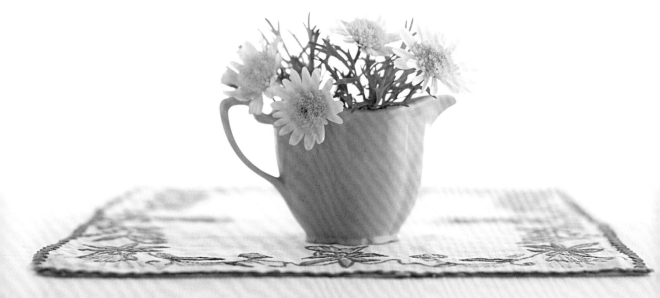

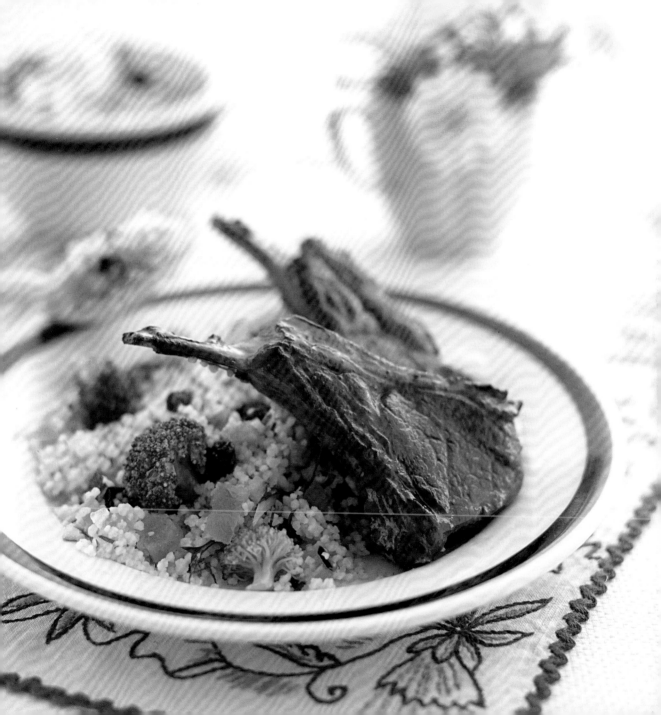

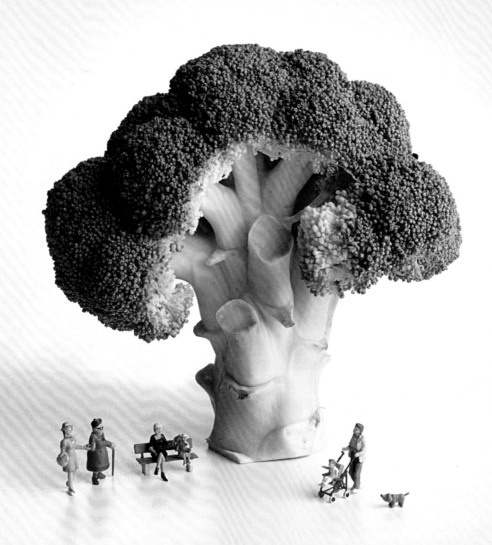

Speedy veggies

Garlic pita breadsticks

Crudités served with delicious homemade breadsticks make wonderful finger food.

SUITABLE FOR FREEZING
MAKES 20 STICKS
4 large pita breads
2 tablespoons butter, softened
1 small garlic clove, crushed
2 tablespoons pesto
¼ heaping cup finely grated Parmesan cheese

◉ Preheat the broiler to high. Arrange the pitas on a baking sheet. Mix the butter, garlic, and pesto. Spread on one side of the pitas.

◉ Sprinkle with the cheese. Broil for 4 to 5 minutes until golden brown and bubbling.

◉ Let cool, then slice into sticks.

Sun-dried tomato sticks

NOT SUITABLE FOR FREEZING
MAKES 20 STICKS
4 large pita breads
¼ heaping cup sun-dried tomato paste, or 4 sun-dried tomatoes (packed in oil), finely chopped
¼ heaping cup finely grated Parmesan cheese

◉ Preheat the broiler to its highest setting. Arrange the pitas on a baking sheet.

◉ Spread the tomato paste on one side. Sprinkle with the cheese and broil for 4 to 5 minutes, until golden and crisp.

◉ Let cool, then slice into sticks.

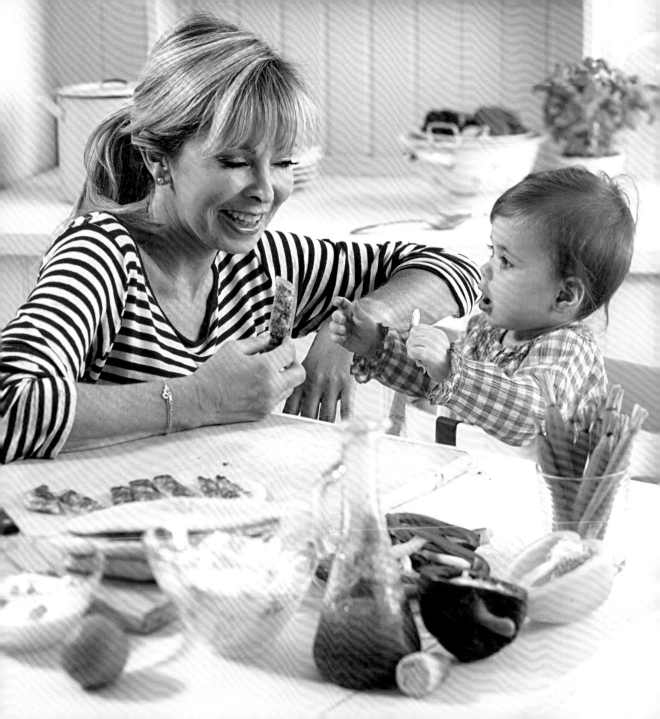

Dips

Serve with cucumber, carrot, bell pepper sticks, pita bread, and cherry tomatoes; or try some more unusual vegetables, such as sugar snap peas, for dipping.

Sweet chili and cream cheese

NOT SUITABLE FOR FREEZING
7 tablespoons light cream cheese (Neufchâtel)
1 teaspoon chopped fresh chives
1 teaspoon sweet chili sauce

⦿ Mix the cream cheese and chives and put in a ramekin. Spoon on the chili sauce, or mix together if you prefer.

Thousand island

NOT SUITABLE FOR FREEZING
2 tablespoons Greek yogurt
2 tablespoons mayonnaise
2 teaspoons ketchup
½ teaspoon lemon juice
1 to 2 drops Worcestershire sauce

Ranch

NOT SUITABLE FOR FREEZING
3 tablespoons sour cream
2 tablespoons mayonnaise
1 teaspoon lime juice (optional)
1 teaspoon chopped fresh cilantro
1 teaspoon chopped fresh chives

Mango and cream cheese

NOT SUITABLE FOR FREEZING
¼ cup light cream cheese (Neufchâtel)
3 tablespoons plain yogurt
1½ tablespoons mango chutney
1 tablespoon lemon juice
Pinch of curry powder

⦿ Mix all the ingredients in a bowl.

⦿ Season to taste and serve with breadsticks.

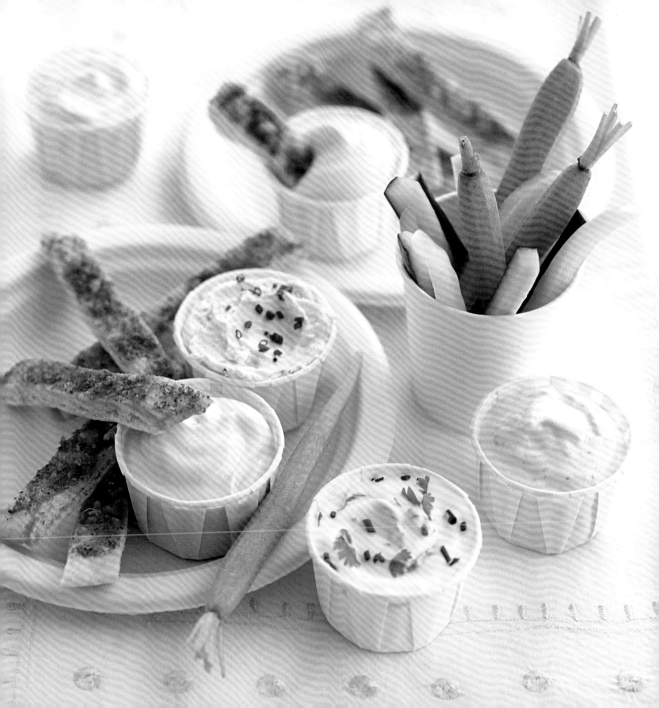

Tomato and cheese quesadilla

20

A few drops of Tabasco add a bit of kick to these quesadillas, but they are still very mild.

NOT SUITABLE FOR FREEZING
MAKES 2 PORTIONS
1 teaspoon canola oil
2 scallions, thinly sliced
8 to 10 cherry tomatoes, coarsely chopped
3 to 4 drops Tabasco
Salt and pepper
2 flour tortillas
½ cup grated Cheddar cheese

◉ Heat the oil in a saucepan or small frying pan. Add the scallions and tomatoes and sauté for 3 to 4 minutes, until the tomatoes are soft.

◉ Remove from the heat and stir in the Tabasco. Season to taste. Heat a large grill pan or nonstick frying pan.

◉ Spread the tomato mixture on one of the tortillas and sprinkle with the cheese.

◉ Cover with the second tortilla and cook in the hot pan for 2 to 3 minutes on each side, until the cheese has melted. Transfer to a cutting board and cut into 12 wedges.

Caramelized onion quesadilla

35

Sweet caramelized onions make a delicious filling for quesadillas.

NOT SUITABLE FOR FREEZING
MAKES 2 PORTIONS
1 tablespoon olive oil
1 large red onion, or 2 small, thinly sliced
½ teaspoon fresh thyme leaves (optional)
1 tablespoon balsamic vinegar
1 teaspoon light brown sugar
Salt and pepper
2 flour tortillas
½ cup grated Cheddar cheese

◉ Heat the oil in a small frying pan. Add the onion and thyme, if using, and cook over medium heat for 15 minutes, until the onion is soft.

◉ Increase the heat to high and add the vinegar and sugar. Cook, stirring until the vinegar has evaporated. Remove from the heat and season to taste. Let cool slightly.

◉ Heat a large nonstick frying pan or grill pan. Spread the onions on one of the tortillas and sprinkle with the cheese.

◉ Cover with the second tortilla, then grill for 2 to 3 minutes on each side, until the cheese has melted, or cook in the frying pan. Transfer to a cutting board and cut into 12 wedges.

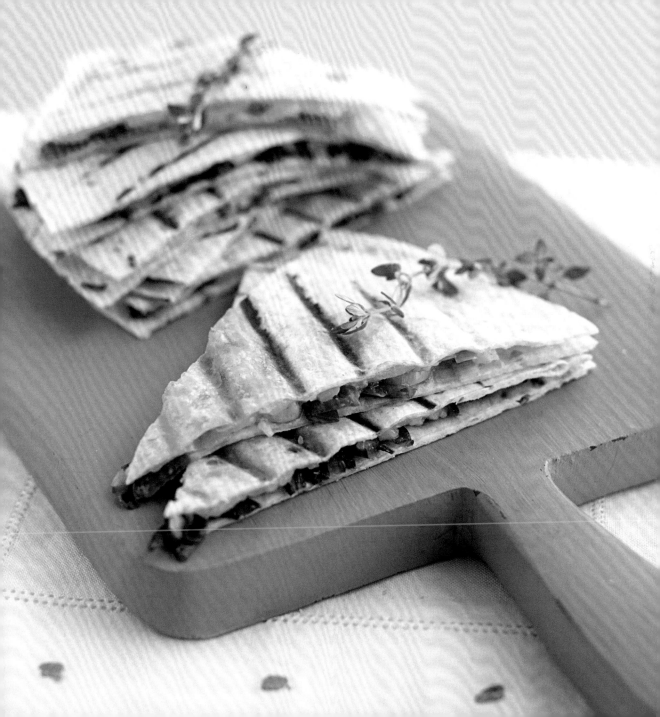

Tasty veggie burrito

This makes the most delicious meal and it's easy to double the quantity. Simply make two separate omelets and just cook double the amount of filling.

1 flour tortilla (about 8-inch diameter)
1 egg
Salt and pepper
1 tablespoon butter
¼ medium red onion, finely chopped
¼ red bell pepper, diced
1 sprig fresh thyme, leaves removed
Pinch of paprika
1 tomato, seeded and diced
2 to 3 drops Tabasco (optional)
¼ cup grated Cheddar cheese
1 tablespoon sour cream (optional)

◉ Put the tortilla on a large plate. Beat the egg with 1 teaspoon of water and a little salt and pepper.

◉ Heat half the butter in a nonstick frying pan. Add the egg and tip the pan to spread out and make a thin omelet. Cook for 2 to 3 minutes, until the omelet has set, then slide it onto the tortilla.

◉ Heat the remaining butter in the frying pan and, when foaming, add the onion, bell pepper, thyme, and paprika and sauté for 5 minutes, or until the onion and pepper are soft. Add the tomato and cook for another 2 minutes, until the tomato is soft.

◉ Add the Tabasco, if using, and season with salt and pepper. Remove the pan from the heat and set aside for a moment.

◉ Heat the tortilla and omelet for 10 to 20 seconds in a microwave, spoon the onion mixture over the center, sprinkle with the cheese, and roll up. Serve immediately with a spoonful of sour cream, if you like.

◉ If you prefer, you can cut the omelet into little strips and mix in with the onion mixture.

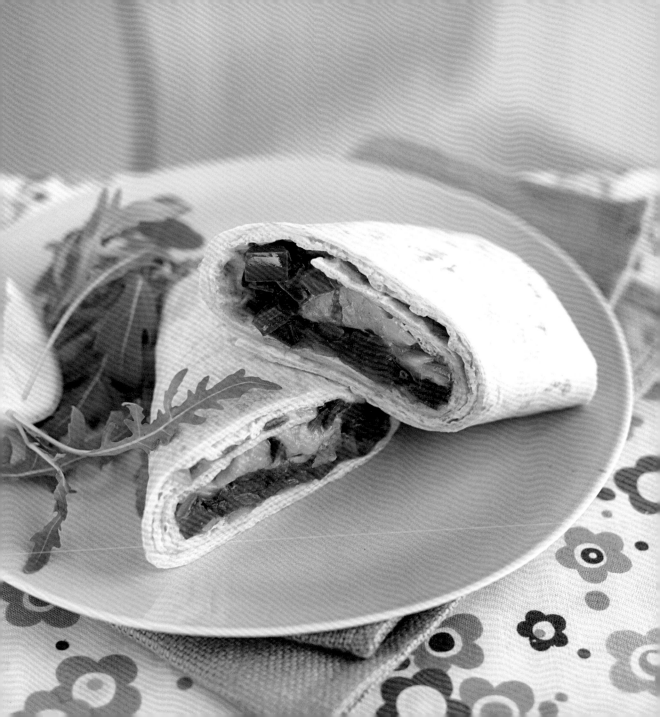

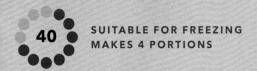

SUITABLE FOR FREEZING
MAKES 4 PORTIONS

Tomato soup

This is a tasty, simple-to-prepare soup.

2 teaspoons olive oil
1 large celery stalk, thinly sliced
1 large onion, finely chopped
1 carrot, grated (about ¾ cup)
1 garlic clove, crushed
1 (14-ounce) can diced tomatoes
1¼ cups vegetable or chicken broth
2 large ripe tomatoes, quartered
1 teaspoon tomato paste
¼ teaspoon brown sugar (optional)

◉ Heat the oil in a saucepan. Add the celery, onion, carrot, and garlic and fry for 5 minutes.

◉ Add the remaining ingredients. Bring to a boil, then simmer for 10 to 15 minutes, covered, until all the vegetables are soft.

◉ Blend with a hand blender until smooth.

Lentil and vegetable soup

Lentils are a good source of protein and iron. A good way to get children to enjoy eating them is to whiz them up with sautéed vegetables to make a delicious soup.

2 teaspoons olive oil
1 medium onion, finely chopped
1 carrot, grated (about ¾ cup)
1 garlic clove, crushed
2 celery stalks, thinly sliced
⅓ cup red lentils
1 cup canned diced tomatoes
2½ cups vegetable broth
1 teaspoon tomato paste
½ teaspoon brown sugar (optional)

◉ Heat the oil in a saucepan on medium heat. Add the onion, carrot, garlic, and celery and fry for 2 to 3 minutes.

◉ Add the lentils and coat in the vegetable mixture. Then add the remaining ingredients.

◉ Bring to a boil, then simmer covered for 20 to 25 minutes, until the vegetables and lentils are soft.

◉ Whiz until smooth with a hand blender.

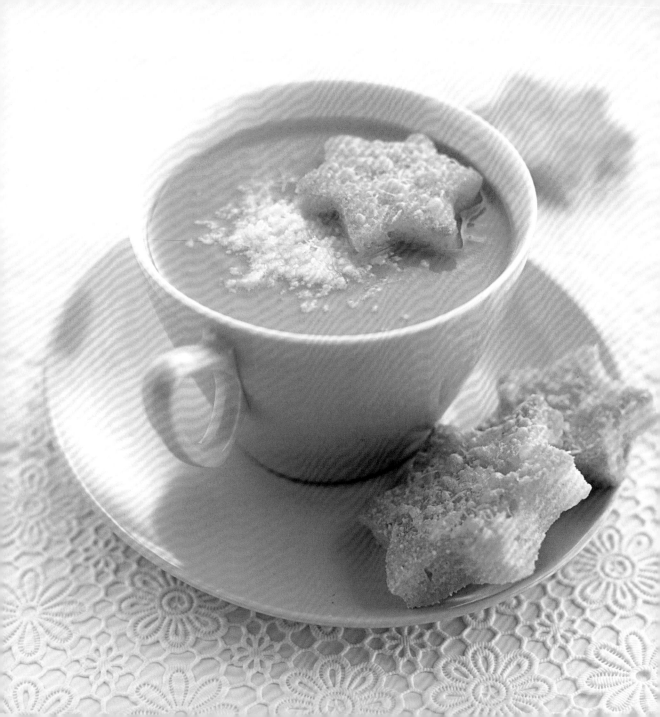

Sweet potato and butternut squash soup with cheesy croutons

This flavorsome soup is enough on its own, but served with cheesy croutons is a real treat.

2 tablespoons olive oil
1 small onion, chopped
½ teaspoon grated fresh ginger
1⅓ cups peeled and diced
    butternut squash
1 cup peeled and diced sweet
    potatoes
1¾ cups chicken broth

For the croutons
2 slices white bread
Olive oil
2 tablespoons finely grated
    Parmesan cheese

◉ Heat the oil in a saucepan on medium heat. Add the onion and ginger and fry for 3 minutes. Add the squash and potatoes.

◉ Fry for 2 minutes, then add the broth. Bring to a boil, then simmer for 15 minutes. Whiz with a hand blender until smooth.

◉ To make the croutons, stamp four stars out of the bread using a star cutter. Lightly brush with oil and sprinkle with the cheese.

◉ Put the croutons onto a baking sheet. Broil for 2 to 3 minutes, until lightly golden. Serve on top of the soup.

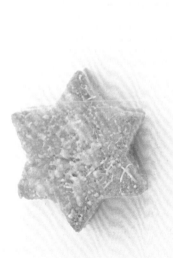
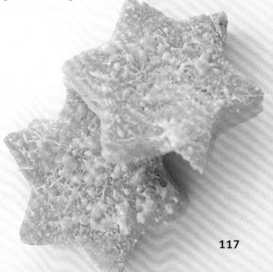

117

Rainbow ribbon noodles

It's fun eating these with child-friendly chopsticks that are joined at the top.

For the omelet
1 tablespoon canola oil
1 egg
1 teaspoon soy sauce
1 teaspoon water

For the noodles
1 small garlic clove, crushed
½ teaspoon grated fresh ginger
1 small carrot, julienned
¼ yellow bell pepper, seeded and
    julienned
½ small zucchini, julienned
3 ounces rice sticks (pad Thai
    noodles) prepared following the
    package directions
2 scallions, thinly sliced
2 teaspoons soy sauce
1 teaspoon sweet chili sauce
½ teaspoon Asian sesame oil
Fresh cilantro, chopped (optional)

◉ Heat 1 teaspoon of the oil in a wok. Beat the egg, soy sauce, and water and add to the wok.

◉ Cook the omelet until just set and brown underneath. Break or chop into pieces and transfer to a bowl. Set aside.

◉ Heat the remaining oil in the wok and add the garlic and ginger. Sauté for 30 seconds, then add the carrot, bell pepper, and zucchini and stir-fry for 3 to 4 minutes, until the vegetables are tender.

◉ Add the noodles and scallions and stir-fry for 1 to 2 minutes, until the noodles have heated through. Stir in the soy sauce, chili sauce, and sesame oil, followed by the omelet pieces, then remove from the heat and transfer to bowls.

◉ Garnish with the cilantro, if you like.

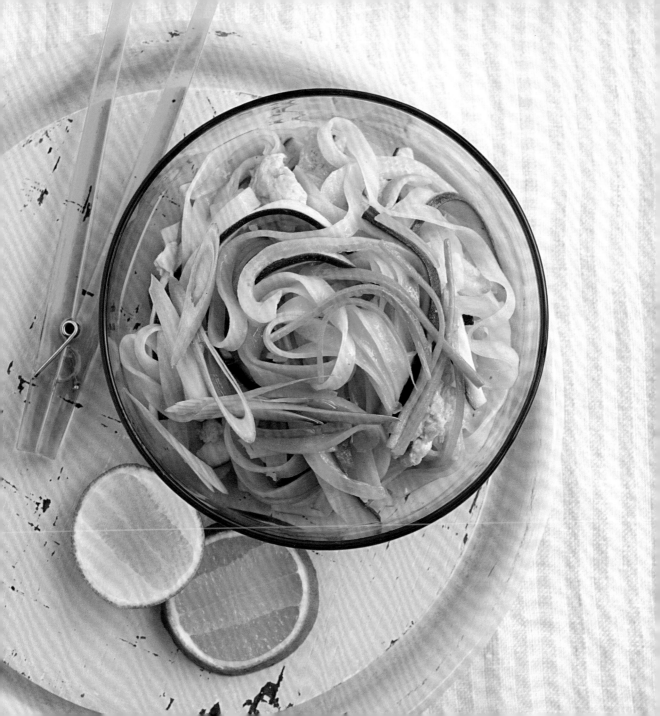

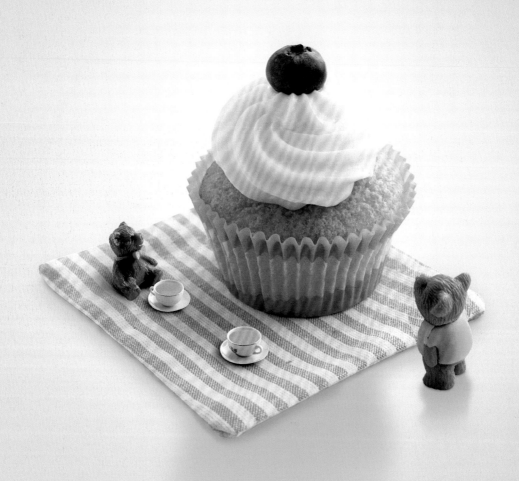

Double-quick desserts and sweet treats

Strawberry and watermelon popsicles

15

A refreshing treat during watermelon season.

MAKES ABOUT 6 SMALL POPSICLES
¼ cup sugar
¼ cup water
2 cups sliced strawberries
1⅔ cups diced seedless watermelon

◉ Put the sugar and water into a small saucepan and boil until syrupy (about 3 minutes). Let cool. Puree the strawberries and strain to remove the seeds.

◉ Puree the watermelon and mix with the strawberries and cooled syrup. Pour the mixture into popsicle molds and freeze.

Lychee popsicles

5

A delicious mix of lychees blended with vanilla yogurt.

MAKES ABOUT 3 POPSICLES
1 (15-ounce) can lychees in syrup, drained
2 tablespoons syrup from the can
¼ cup vanilla yogurt (whole milk)
1 tablespoon lime juice

◉ Whiz the ingredients together, until fairly smooth. Pour into popsicle molds and freeze overnight.

Strawberry and lime popsicles

5

The lime adds a nice zesty taste.

MAKES 4 LARGE POPSICLES
8 ounces strawberries
3 tablespoons Rose's lime juice
2 tablespoons confectioners' sugar

◉ Puree the strawberries, lime juice, and sugar and strain.

◉ Pour into popsicle molds and freeze.

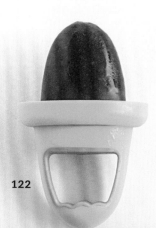

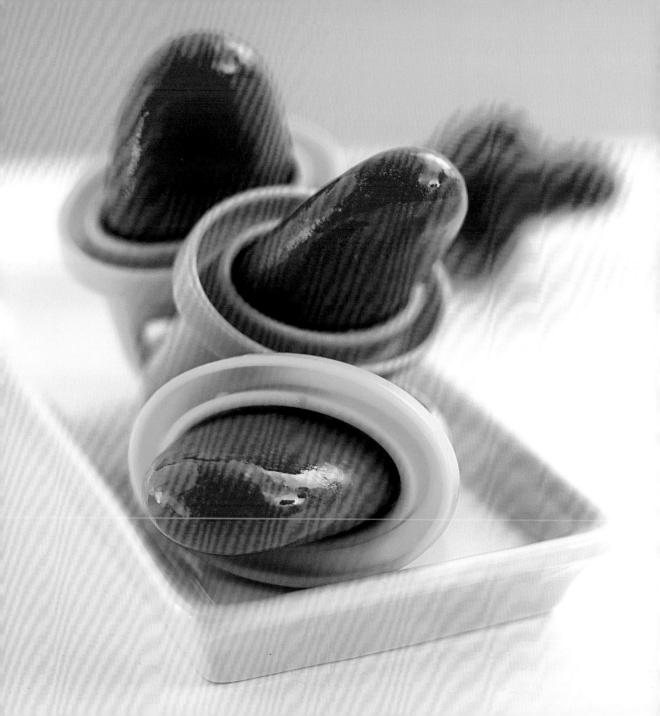

Lemon cupcakes

Children love to help pipe the frosting on cupcakes, so get them involved!

Cupcakes
8 tablespoons (1 stick) unsalted
  butter, at room temperature
1 cup superfine sugar
2 large eggs
1¼ cups self-rising flour, sifted
1 cup all-purpose flour, sifted
½ teaspoon baking powder
⅔ cup low-fat milk
1 teaspoon grated lemon zest

Frosting
2 cups confectioners' sugar
6 tablespoons unsalted butter, at
  room temperature
1 tablespoon lemon juice
2 tablespoons cream cheese

◉ Preheat the oven to 350°F. Line a muffin pan with 12 paper cupcake cases.

◉ To make the cupcakes, put all the cake ingredients into a bowl. Whisk until smooth.

◉ Spoon the mixture into the cupcake cases until two-thirds full. Bake for about 25 minutes until the cupcakes are raised and lightly golden. To check if they are done you can insert a skewer or toothpick into the center of one of the cakes and it should come out clean. Remove the cupcakes from the oven and let cool a little and then arrange the cupcakes on a wire rack to cool completely.

◉ To make the frosting, sift the confectioners' sugar and gradually beat it into the butter using an electric mixer, until smooth. Slowly beat in the lemon juice and cream cheese. Chill until needed. Spread the frosting on top of the cupcake using a spatula, or pipe the frosting on top of each of the cupcakes with a pastry bag.

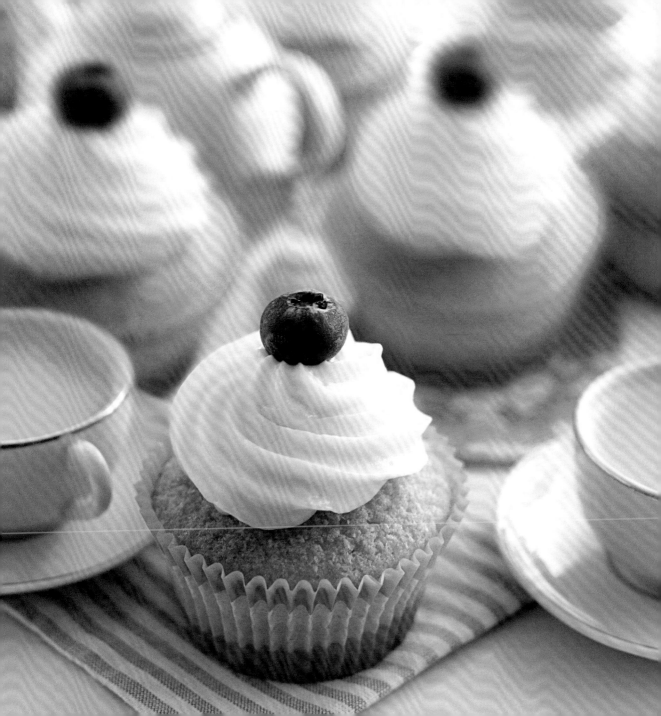

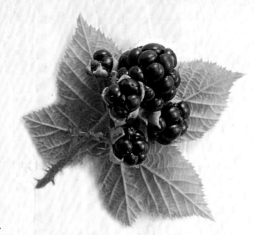

Fruit compote

You can serve this either for breakfast or dessert.

3 apples, peeled, cored, and
    quartered
¼ cup sugar plus extra to taste
1 (16-ounce) package frozen
    mixed berries

◉ Cut each apple quarter into four pieces. Put the apples in a large saucepan with 2 tablespoons of water and the sugar.

◉ Heat gently, stirring occasionally until the sugar has melted. Cover and cook for 8 minutes, until the apples are tender but not mushy.

◉ Add the berries and cook for 5 to 6 minutes more, until the mixture just comes to a boil. Immediately remove from the heat and let cool slightly.

◉ Taste and add more sugar if necessary. Serve warm or chilled.

Variations
◉ Once chilled, the compote can be layered in glasses with yogurt and granola, or put in ovenproof dishes.

◉ Whip heavy cream with 1 teaspoon of confectioners' sugar and 2 to 3 drops of vanilla extract. Fold in 3 tablespoons of Greek yogurt and spoon on the fruit. Sprinkle 1 tablespoon of raw sugar over each and broil until the sugar has melted. You will need to drain most of the liquid, which you could serve separately in a small pitcher.

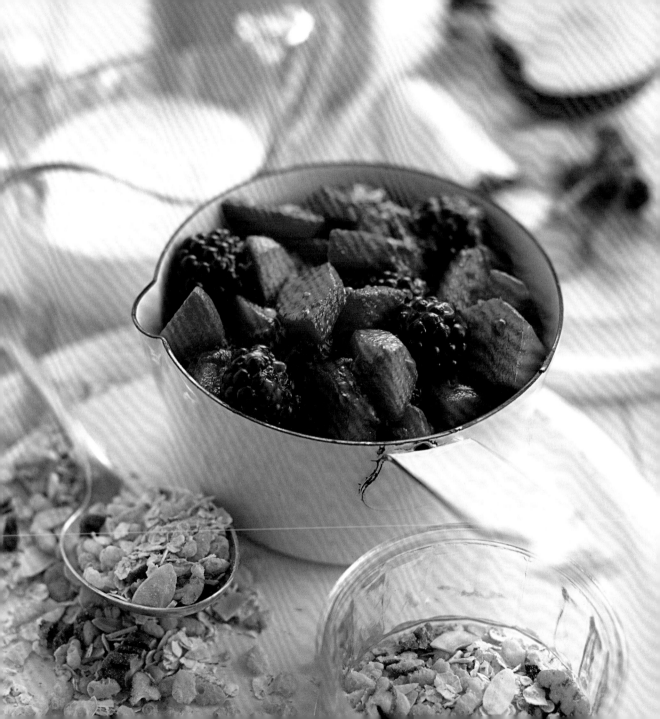

Frozen berry smoothie

You can either buy a bag of frozen berries or freeze some fresh berries overnight.

MAKES 2 GLASSES
1¼ cups (about 5 ounces) frozen berries (raspberries, blackberries, blueberries, or strawberries)
1 small banana
¼ cup strawberry drinking yogurt
7 tablespoons cream soda

◉ Put the frozen berries and banana into a blender and whiz until smooth. Strain into a bowl. Add the yogurt and cream soda and stir. Pour into chilled glasses and serve.

Strawberry and banana smoothie

Choose a ripe banana and sweet strawberries for this smoothie. I prefer to use natural apple juice.

MAKES 2 GLASSES
1 large banana
1¼ cups sliced strawberries
7 tablespoons apple juice

◉ Put the banana, strawberries, and apple juice into a blender and whiz until smooth. Pour into two chilled glasses. Add ice cubes.

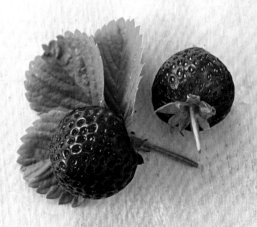

Strawberry sorbet

If you don't have an ice cream maker, freeze in a plastic container and soften, then whiz a couple of times in a food processor until smooth.

MAKES 4 PORTIONS
3¼ cups sliced strawberries
7 tablespoons water
½ cup strawberry or raspberry preserves
½ cup sugar
¼ cup Greek yogurt

◉ Put the strawberries, water, preserves, and sugar in a saucepan. Heat gently until the sugar has melted, then bring to a boil and cook for 1 minute.

◉ Remove from the heat, cool, blend, and strain to remove the seeds. Stir in the yogurt and chill.

◉ Churn in an ice cream maker until frozen.

Banana bread

This is delicious for breakfast or as a snack. It's best made with very ripe bananas. It's lovely and moist, and keeps very well.

SUITABLE FOR FREEZING
MAKES 8 PORTIONS
1 pound ripe bananas
8 tablespoons (1 stick) butter, at room temperature
⅔ cup light brown sugar
1¾ cups self-rising flour
1 egg
¼ cup low-fat yogurt
1 teaspoon vanilla extract
¾ cup raisins

◉ Preheat the oven to 350°F.

◉ Line a two pound loaf pan with parchment paper.

◉ Put the bananas in a food processor and whiz for about 30 seconds, until coarsely chopped. Add the butter, brown sugar, flour, egg, yogurt, and vanilla and whiz for 1 to 2 minutes, until combined into a smooth batter. Add the raisins.

◉ Spoon into the loaf pan. Bake for 1 hour, until a toothpick inserted into the center comes out clean. Cool in the pan for 30 minutes, then remove the loaf from the pan and cool completely on a wire rack.

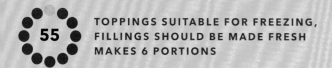
Crumble jumble

When babies first move from purees to soft foods it is useful to have some flavors that are familiar, such as blueberries, apples, and pears. The fruit in crumbles is soft enough to be munched by gums, but not so soft that it is a puree. Older children and grown-ups also love crumbles. Here I have given you three different toppings and three different fillings, which you can mix and match as you like—there are nine possible combinations! The quantities are for a large crumble baked in an 8-inch round baking pan (6 cups capacity), or six ramekins (7 ounces capacity).

● ● ● ● ● ● ● ● ● ● ● ● ● ●

TIP
If you are making a crumble topping, try making a double quantity and freezing half in a resealable bag. You can sprinkle the topping directly over the fruit base.

TOPPINGS
Classic crumble

⅔ cup all-purpose flour
3 tablespoons butter, cut into cubes
¼ cup sugar
¾ teaspoon cinnamon
¼ teaspoon salt

Ginger oat

⅔ cup all-purpose flour
¼ cup quick-cooking oats (not instant)
3 tablespoons butter, cut into cubes
½ teaspoon ground ginger
Pinch of salt
¼ cup light brown sugar

Flaky almond

⅔ cup all-purpose flour
¼ cup sliced almonds plus an extra
    ¼ cup for optional topping
3 tablespoons butter, cut into cubes
¼ cup sugar
¼ teaspoon ground cinnamon

Whiz the ingredients in a food processor until large crumbs form that look like rolled oats. Sprinkle over the fruit.

Optional: Sprinkle the extra sliced almonds over the crumble for the last 10 minutes of the cooking time.

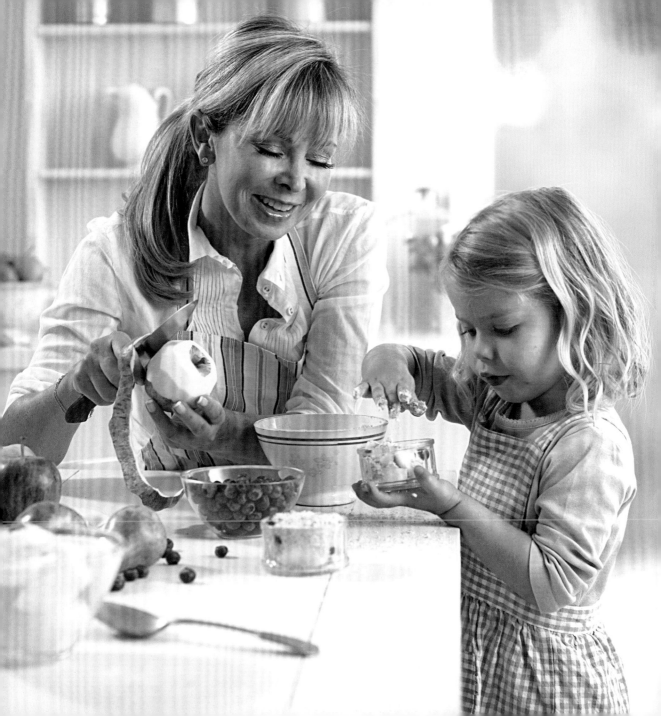

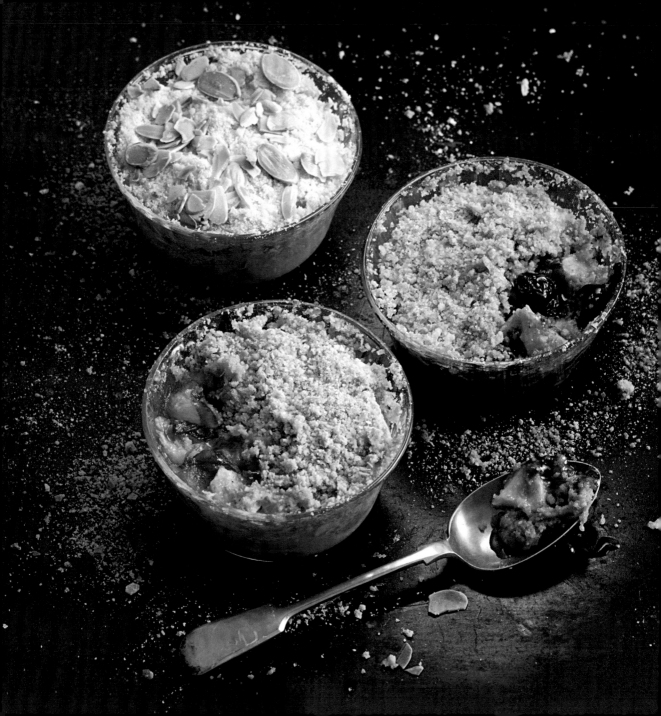

Rhubarb and apple

2 large Granny Smith apples (about 14 ounces)
   peeled, cored, and diced
10 ounces rhubarb, trimmed and cut into
   ⅜ inch-pieces
½ cup sugar

◉ Preheat the oven to 400°F. Toss the apples, rhubarb, and sugar together in the dish. Sprinkle with your chosen topping and bake for 35 to 40 minutes, until the topping is golden brown and the juices of the fruit are bubbling. For individual crumbles bake for 25 to 30 minutes.

Apple and blueberry

2⅓ cups blueberries
2 large Granny Smith apples (about 14 ounces),
   peeled, cored, and diced
Zest of 1 lemon (optional)
¼ cup sugar

◉ Preheat the oven to 400°F. Toss the blueberries, apples, lemon zest, if using, and sugar in the dish. Sprinkle with your chosen topping and bake for 35 to 40

minutes, until the topping is golden brown and the juices of the fruit are bubbling. For individual crumbles bake for 25 to 30 minutes.

Orchard fruits

2 apples, peeled, cored, and diced
2 large pears, peeled, cored, and diced
4 teaspoons sugar, or to taste

◉ Preheat the oven to 400°F. Put the fruit in a small saucepan and simmer for 10 to 15 minutes, until it is soft but not mushy.

◉ Remove the fruit from the heat and stir in the sugar, adding more if the fruit isn't sweet enough.

◉ Transfer to the baking dish, sprinkle with your chosen topping, and bake for 30 minutes, until the topping is golden brown. For individual crumbles bake for 25 minutes.

Annabel's oat bars

NOT SUITABLE FOR FREEZING
MAKES 12 BARS
6 tablespoons butter
½ cup light brown sugar
3 tablespoons corn syrup
1 cup quick-cooking oats (not instant)
1 cup Rice Krispies
¼ teaspoon salt
½ cup unsweetened shredded coconut
⅓ cup chopped dried apricots
¼ cup cranberries
¼ cup raisins
¼ cup chopped pecans (optional)

◉ Preheat the oven to 325° F.

◉ Line an 8 inch-square pan with parchment paper, with the parchment coming up the sides.

◉ Put the butter, sugar, and corn syrup in a large saucepan.

◉ Heat gently, stirring occasionally, until butter and sugar have melted. Remove from the heat and mix in the remaining ingredients. Spoon into the prepared pan and spread in an even layer (a potato masher is useful). Bake for 25 minutes, until golden around the edges. Cool completely in the pan, then lift out and cut into 12 small bars. You may need to store these in the fridge.

Chocolate and apricot Rice Krispie squares

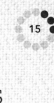

NOT SUITABLE FOR FREEZING
MAKES 9 SQUARES
5 tablespoons butter
¼ cup corn syrup
⅓ cup semisweet chocolate chips
⅔ cup quick-cooking oats (not instant)
2 cups Rice Krispies
½ cup chopped dried apricots or mixture
   of dried exotic fruits

◉ Put the butter, corn syrup, and chocolate chips into a medium saucepan and heat gently until melted.

◉ Combine the oats, Rice Krispies, and apricots in a mixing bowl.

◉ Remove from the heat. Pour the dry ingredients into the chocolate mixture and stir until well coated.

◉ Spread the mixture in an 8 inch-square shallow baking pan and store in the fridge. Cut into squares and store them there until ready to serve.

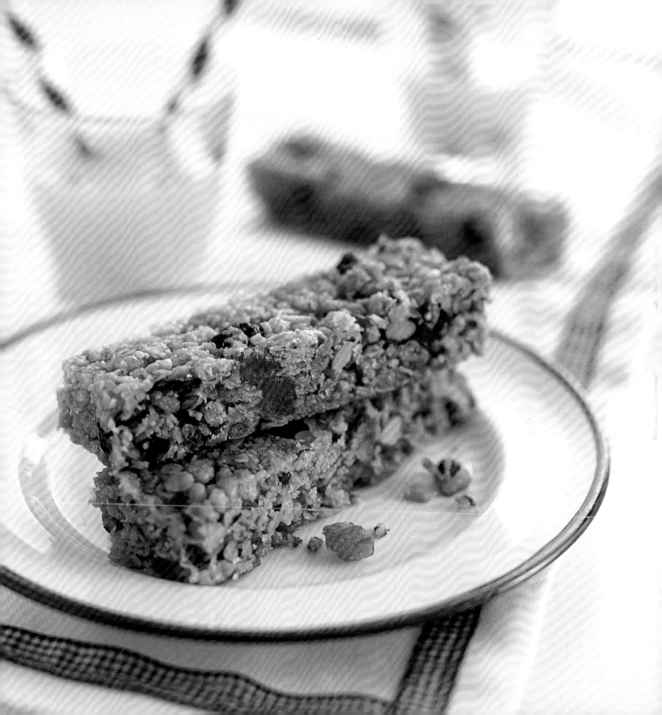

Chocolate zucchini muffins

SUITABLE FOR FREEZING
MAKES 10 LARGE OR 24 MINI MUFFINS
1½ cups all-purpose flour
2 teaspoons baking powder
¾ cup light brown sugar
2 tablespoons unsweetened cocoa powder
1¼ cups grated zucchini
Zest of 1 small orange (optional)
½ cup canola oil
1 egg, beaten
¼ cup Greek yogurt or plain yogurt (whole milk)
1 teaspoon vanilla extract
¼ cup milk chocolate chips

◉ Preheat the oven to 350°F. Line a standard muffin pan with 10 paper cases or a mini muffin pan with 24 paper cases.

◉ Put the flour, baking powder, sugar, cocoa, zucchini, and zest into a mixing bowl.

◉ Put the oil, egg, yogurt, and vanilla into a cup and whisk together.

◉ Add the wet ingredients to the dry and mix until smooth. Stir in the chocolate chips. Divide the mixture between the muffin cases. Bake the large muffins for 20 to 25 minutes, the mini muffins for about 14 minutes, until the muffins are well risen and springy to the touch. Cool on a wire rack.

Carrot, apple, and golden raisin muffins

SUITABLE FOR FREEZING
MAKES 12 MUFFINS
1⅔ cups self-rising flour
1 teaspoon baking powder
¾ teaspoon baking soda
1½ teaspoons pumpkin pie spice
½ teaspoon ground ginger
¾ cup canola oil
½ cup superfine sugar
2 eggs
1 cup grated carrots
1 cup peeled and grated apple
½ cup golden raisins

◉ Preheat the oven to 350° F. Line a standard muffin pan with 12 paper cases.

◉ Put all the ingredients into a bowl. Whisk using an electric hand mixer, until blended. Divide between the paper cases.

◉ Bake for 18 to 20 minutes, until golden and well risen.

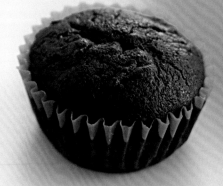

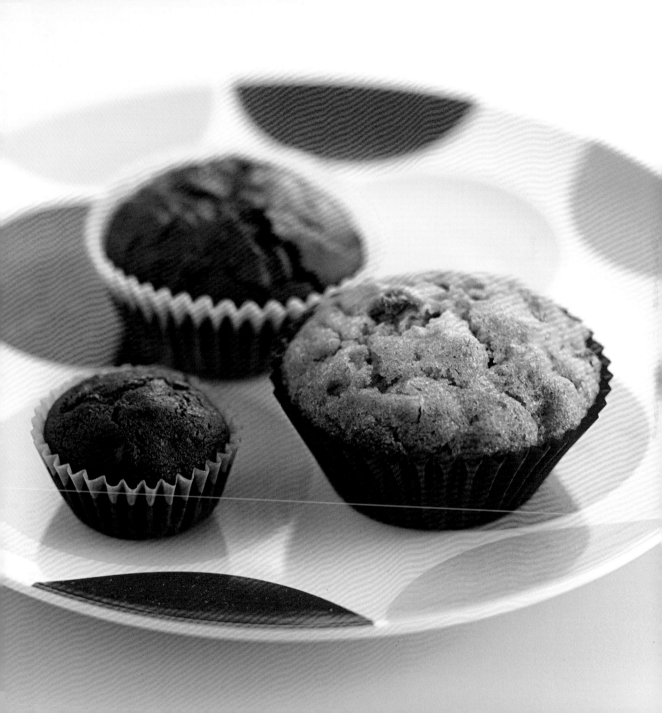

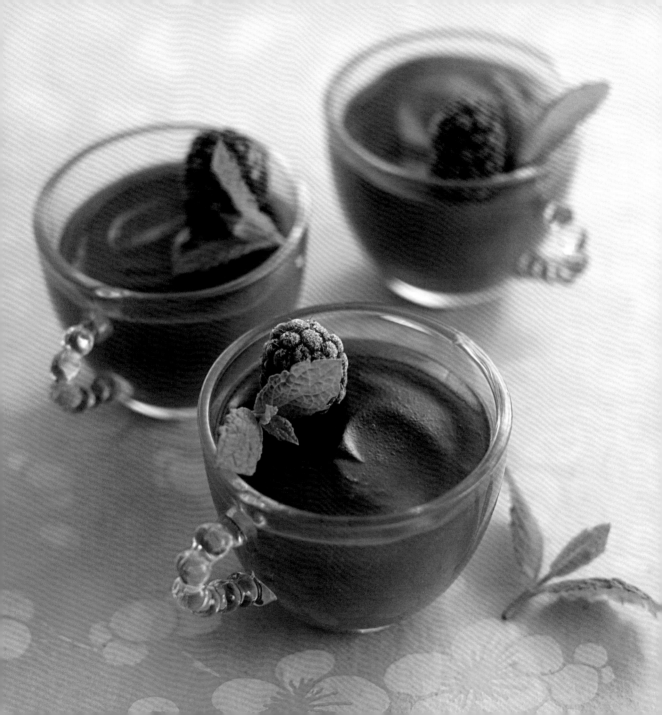

Chocolate self-saucing sponge

55

NOT SUITABLE FOR FREEZING
MAKES 6 PORTIONS

For the chocolate sponge
3 tablespoons soft butter plus extra for greasing
¼ cup light brown sugar
¾ cup self-rising flour
3 tablespoons unsweetened cocoa powder
⅓ cup milk
1 egg
½ teaspoon vanilla extract
Pinch of salt
3 tablespoons semisweet chocolate chips

For the sauce
½ cup light brown sugar
2 tablespoons unsweetened cocoa powder
1 teaspoon instant coffee granules
¾ cup boiling water

◉ Preheat the oven to 325°F. Grease a 6 cup capacity deep baking dish. Put all the sponge ingredients, except the chocolate chips, in a food processor and whiz for 1 to 2 minutes to combine. Add the chocolate chips and pulse 4 to 5 times to distribute. Scrape the batter into the prepared dish.

◉ Whisk the sauce ingredients in an ovenproof bowl or cup and pour over the sponge batter. Bake for 35 to 40 minutes, until the sponge has risen and a skewer inserted into the center comes out without any raw batter on it. The sauce will also be bubbling up the sides of the sponge. Serve with vanilla ice cream.

Creamy chocolate pots

25

NOT SUITABLE FOR FREEZING
MAKES 4 SMALL POTS
1¼ cups whole milk
¼ cup heavy cream
2 egg yolks
4 teaspoons cornstarch
⅓ cup superfine sugar
¼ cup bittersweet chocolate chips
½ teaspoon vanilla extract
Pat of butter

◉ Put the milk and cream in a saucepan. Heat gently until almost boiling. Meanwhile, put the egg yolks, cornstarch, and sugar in a bowl and whisk.

◉ Pour the hot milk and cream into the egg mixture in a thin stream, whisking constantly. Rinse the saucepan to remove any milk from the base. Then pour the custard into the pan and cook over medium-low heat, whisking or stirring constantly, until the custard just comes up to a boil and thickens. Remove from the heat and whisk in the chocolate, vanilla, and butter.

◉ Pour into four small ramekins and chill for 5 to 6 hours (or overnight) until set. You can press a piece of plastic wrap onto the surface of each chocolate cup if you want to prevent a skin from forming.

Index

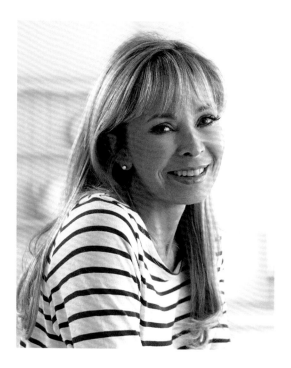

outstanding work in the field of child nutrition, Annabel was awarded an MBE (Member of the British Empire) in the Queen's Birthday Honours in 2006.

Passionate about improving the way children eat, Annabel has designed healthy children's menus for some of the world's largest hotels and leisure resorts. Annabel's sought-after recipes have also grown into a successful supermarket food line, including purees, snacks, and toddler meals.

Annabel is a regular commentator in the media on health and food issues. Her US highlights include appearing on the *Today* show and writing for leading parenting publications including Parents.com and Babycenter.com.

Books are not the only string to Annabel's bow (or should we say apron!); she has developed a bestselling app (*Annabel's Essential Guide to Feeding Your Baby and Toddler*) which has been extremely popular with parents in the United States, and her website www.annabelkarmel.com attracts more than 3.6 million users annually.

Annabel is also recognized as a leading female entrepreneur and has become an inspirational role model for women—especially mothers—who want to set up in business and have thriving careers while raising a family.

Twenty-five years since coming to the rescue of parents with her very first weaning guide, Annabel Karmel has changed the eating habits of millions of babies and children across the world.

Mother of three, Annabel, is the United Kingdom's number one children's cookery author, bestselling international author, and leading expert on feeding growing families with thirty-eight books selling four million copies worldwide. Annabel's very first book, *The Healthy Baby Meal Planner,* is the second bestselling nonfiction hardcover of all time.

From first foods to family meals, Annabel continues to be the United Kingdom's most trusted, influential, and inspiring resource for parents who want to give their growing family the very best start in life. In fact, for her

annabel karmel   **www.annabelkarmel.com**

ACKNOWLEDGMENTS

I would like to thank the following for their help and work on this book: Dave King for his excellent photography; Smith & Gilmour for their beautiful design; food stylist Seiko Hatfield; Lucinda McCord; Jo Harris for her props styling; the team at Atria, including Judith Curr, Greer Hendricks, Sarah Cantin, Dana Sloan, Stacey Kulig, Kimberly Goldstein, Kristen Lemire, Ben Lee, Elaine Broeder, and Jackie Jou; Caroline Stearns; Helena Caldon; and Jo Godfrey Wood.

Last but by no means least, I would like to thank my children, Nicholas, Lara, and Scarlett, for tasting all my recipes.

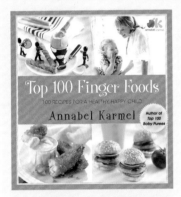

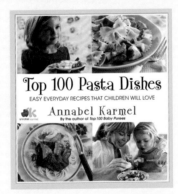

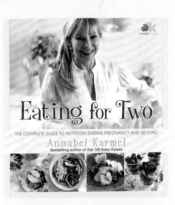

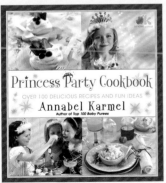

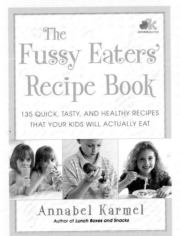

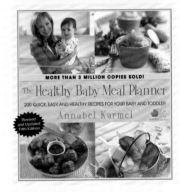

Recipes at your fingertips!

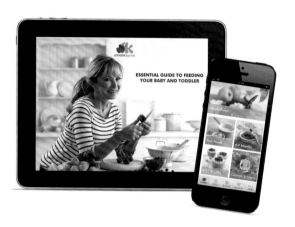

For lots more recipe inspiration for your growing family, check out **Annabel's Essential Guide to Feeding Your Baby and Toddler** app.

With instant access to more than 200 delicious, easy-to-follow recipes, as well as a host of features including weekly planners, shopping lists, a kitchen timer, and recipe videos, it's the ultimate guide to help you shop for, prep, and cook delicious food for your growing family. Available from the App Store.

Top 100 Baby Purees

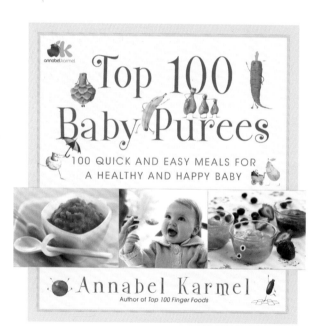

Weaning can be a tricky milestone, especially if you don't have time to spend countless hours in the kitchen preparing and experimenting with new ingredients.

Bestselling parenting author, Annabel Karmel MBE, has done the hard work for moms and dads with **Top 100 Baby Purees.** Using her wealth of experience and expertise in feeding babies, her handy book is filled with 100 fast, tasty, and nutritious recipes.

From first tastes to introducing more adventurous flavors and textures, Annabel is on hand to help families raise healthy, happy babies.

www.annabelkarmel.com
Facebook: **annabelkarmeluk**
Twitter: @annabelkarmel